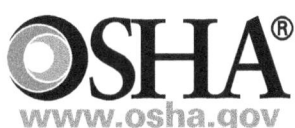
www.osha.gov

Occupational Safety and Health Act of 1970

"To assure safe and healthful working conditions for working men and women; by authorizing enforcement of the standards developed under the Act; by assisting and encouraging the States in their efforts to assure safe and healthful working conditions; by providing for research, information, education, and training in the field of occupational safety and health."

Material contained in this publication is in the public domain and may be reproduced, fully or partially, without permission. Source credit is requested but not required.

This information will be made available to sensory-impaired individuals upon request.
Voice phone: (202) 693-1999;
teletypewriter (TTY) number: 1-877-889-5627.

This publication provides a general overview of a particular standards-related topic. This publication does not alter or determine compliance responsibilities which are set forth in OSHA standards, and the *Occupational Safety and Health Act.* Moreover, because interpretations and enforcement policy may change over time, for additional guidance on OSHA compliance requirements, the reader should consult current administrative interpretations and decisions by the Occupational Safety and Health Review Commission and the courts.

OSHA would like to thank the American College of Occupational and Environmental Medicine (ACOEM) and M.C. Townsend Associates, LLC for their assistance in preparing this document.

Cover photo courtesy of Vitalograph. This image is for informational purposes only and does not represent an official OSHA endorsement of the products shown or their manufacturer.

Spirometry Testing in Occupational Health Programs

Best Practices for Healthcare Professionals

**Occupational Safety and Health Administration
U.S. Department of Labor**

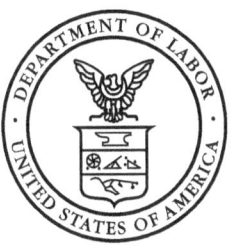

OSHA 3637-03 2013

TABLE OF CONTENTS

1.0 INTRODUCTION 1

    1.1 SPIROMETRY OVERVIEW 2

2.0 ACCURATELY MEASURING WORKER LUNG FUNCTION...3

    2.1 PERSONNEL INVOLVED IN SPIROMETRY TESTING 3

    2.2 EQUIPMENT 5

    2.3 CONDUCTING SPIROMETRY TESTS 16

3.0 INTERPRETING TEST RESULTS 28

    3.1 COMPARING WORKER RESULTS WITH THE NORMAL RANGE
    (REFERENCE VALUES) 28

    3.2 EVALUATING RESULTS OVER TIME 32

4.0 QUALITY ASSURANCE (QA) REVIEWS 35

5.0 SPIROMETRY PROCEDURE MANUAL..36

6.0 RECORDKEEPING 37

7.0 REFERENCES 38

APPENDIX A: NATIONAL HEALTH AND NUTRITION EXAMINATION SURVEY III
(NHANES III) REFERENCE VALUES 40

APPENDIX B: CHECKLIST FOR SPIROMETRY PROCEDURE MANUAL 54

OSHA REGIONAL OFFICES..56

HOW TO CONTACT OSHA 57

1.0 INTRODUCTION

Spirometry, the most common type of pulmonary function test (PFT), is used to evaluate worker respiratory health in medical surveillance programs and to screen workers for their ability to perform certain tasks. Spirometry results can play a central role in decisions about worker job assignments and personal protective equipment, and in the assessment of exposure-related health effects. OSHA standards for asbestos, cadmium, coke oven emissions, and cotton dust require spirometry testing as part of medical surveillance (see 29 CFR 1910.1001, 1910.1027, 1910.1029, and 1910.1043). OSHA standards for formaldehyde and benzene require pulmonary function testing when respiratory protection is used at work (see 29 CFR 1910.1048 and 1910.1028).

Whether spirometry is conducted to comply with an OSHA regulation or as part of another workplace-mandated program, its value is compromised when testing is conducted incorrectly, equipment is inaccurate, or results are misinterpreted. Technically flawed tests too often lead to inaccurate interpretations of worker respiratory health, falsely labeling normal subjects as "impaired" or impaired subjects as "normal." Such flawed test results are not only useless but also convey false information which could be harmful to workers (1). Too often, those who conduct the tests or interpret the results are unaware of the impact of technical pitfalls and of current spirometry testing recommendations.

Because spirometry has become so important in occupational health practice, OSHA developed this guidance document to summarize what it regards as the elements of a good occupational health spirometry program. Recommendations are based on current guidelines from the American Thoracic Society/European Respiratory Society (ATS/ERS), the American College of Occupational and Environmental Medicine (ACOEM), and the National Institute for Occupational Safety and Health (NIOSH) (2–8). OSHA's goal is to provide an update for the medical community on what are the required components for valid tests and strategies for interpreting results, so that occupational spirometry tests are useable and of high technical quality.

This document provides a brief overview of the elements of spirometry, followed by specific recommendations on: (1) accurate measurement of worker lung function (training of personnel, equipment considerations, and spirometry test procedures); (2) appropriate interpretation of valid tests (comparing worker results with normal reference values and evaluating worker results over time); (3) Quality Assurance (QA) reviews; and (4) recordkeeping. This document is organized to permit all readers, regardless of their level of spirometry experience, to refer immediately to specific sections of interest.

PURPOSE OF THIS GUIDE

This guidance document is intended for medical personnel who oversee worker health programs, conduct spirometry tests, and/or interpret spirometry results. The goal of the document is to help ensure the collection of accurate, valid spirometry results that are interpreted correctly. Such spirometry assessments can be used to make well-informed decisions about worker respiratory health (including the need for medical referrals), and to conduct programs for prevention and early intervention.

1.1 SPIROMETRY OVERVIEW

Some respiratory diseases slow the speed of expired air; others reduce the volume of air that can be inspired and then exhaled. To detect these impairments, spirometry measures the maximal volume and speed of air that is forcibly exhaled after taking a maximal inspiration. Forced Vital Capacity (FVC) is defined as total exhaled volume after full inspiration. Speed of expired air is determined by dividing the volume of air exhaled in the first second, i.e., the Forced Expiratory Volume in One Second (FEV_1), by the total FVC to give the FEV_1/FVC ratio. The time course of the expiration is recorded as a volume-time curve, and changes in expiratory flow rate are shown as a flow-volume curve (Figure 1).

Measurements from a worker's valid spirometry test are compared with a normal range (i.e., reference values) and/or with that worker's baseline test results to determine whether the measured volume and flow rate are significantly smaller or slower than expected. As described below, both the spirometry test itself and the comparison of results with the normal range and/or baseline values should be performed carefully to guarantee an accurate interpretation of a worker's respiratory health. This document focuses first on accurately measuring worker lung function and second on appropriately interpreting test results. Recommendations are also made regarding QA review programs and recordkeeping.

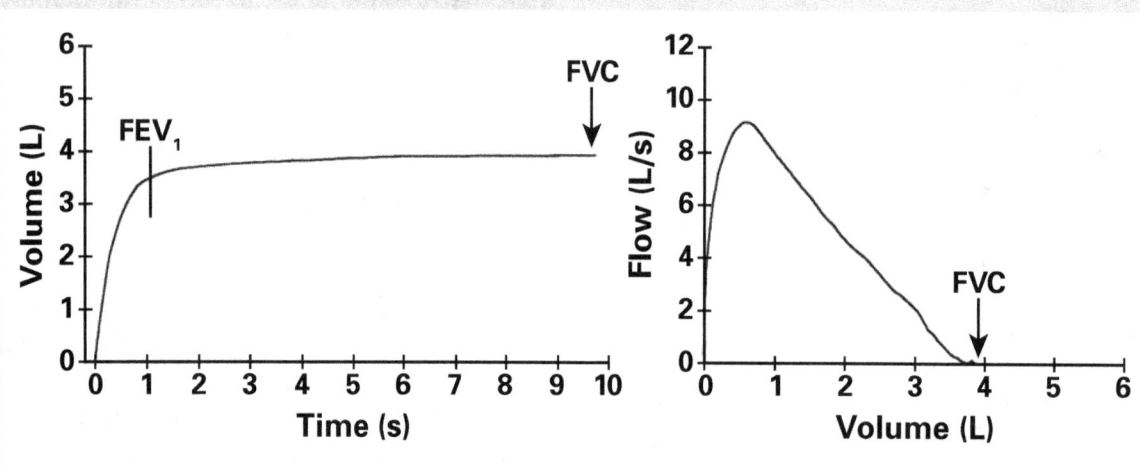

Figure 1. **Volume-time curve (left) and flow-volume curve (right).**

Reproduced with permission from ACOEM (5).

2.0 ACCURATELY MEASURING WORKER LUNG FUNCTION

Three factors work together to produce accurate, meaningful test results: (1) the technician should be well-trained, supervised, and skilled to coach the worker to record optimal test results; (2) the spirometer should be accurate; and (3) the worker should perform with maximal effort and cooperation. Failure of any one of these factors (e.g., the technician has poor coaching skills, equipment is inaccurate, or a worker does not perform maximal efforts) is likely to produce inaccurate results and lead to an incorrect assessment of respiratory health.

2.1 PERSONNEL INVOLVED IN SPIROMETRY TESTING

Medical personnel who conduct spirometry tests and/or interpret the results should be able to identify technically flawed curves and distinguish valid from invalid tests. Commonly used spirometers generate printouts and reports, regardless of whether results are accurate. Simply reading a spirometer's interpretation is insufficient and can lead to serious misclassification of respiratory health if tests are invalid. Training, knowledge, and understanding of spirometry pitfalls are essential for all medical personnel involved in occupational spirometry testing programs.

Occupational spirometry tests are performed by healthcare personnel with varied backgrounds and credentials, ranging from physicians to medical assistants. Generally, the two types of personnel involved in spirometry testing and their responsibilities can be described as follows:

(1) *Physician or Other Licensed Health Care Professional (PLHCP).* In this document, the term PLHCP includes physicians, physician assistants, nurse practitioners, and in some workplaces, registered nurses. PLHCPs often oversee the occupational spirometry program, supervise technicians, clinically interpret spirometry screening test results, and evaluate grouped spirometry data for medical surveillance purposes. The PLHCP may be responsible for ensuring that technicians are well-trained and maintain their levels of competency, have the resources to do their job properly, and follow the clinic's spirometry program guidelines. In some cases, the PLCHP may also conduct spirometry tests. The PLHCP should be able to: (a) evaluate the technical quality and validity of spirometry results before determining whether they indicate normal or impaired respiratory function; (b) communicate the meaning of the test results to the worker who was tested; and (c) evaluate test results for groups of workers at a workplace to determine if patterns of abnormal lung function might indicate a hazardous workplace exposure.

(2) *Technicians.* Spirometry technicians play a critical role in obtaining accurate and precise results. They often have primary responsibility for maintaining the spirometer and checking its accuracy, preparing and coaching workers during testing, and determining whether tests are valid. Motivation to effectively test each worker and the ability to recognize and correct testing errors are essential qualities in a technician.

> OSHA states: "The most important quality of a pulmonary function technician is the motivation to do the very best test on every employee. The technician must also be able to judge the degree of effort and cooperation of the subject. The test results obtained by a technician who lacks these skills are not only useless, but also convey false information which could be harmful to the employee." (1)

2.1.1 TRAINING

Since clinical training programs do not emphasize recognition and troubleshooting of spirometry technical errors, the National Institute for Occupational Safety and Health (NIOSH) approves courses that emphasize how to conduct accurate spirometry tests. The 2–3 day courses cover the fundamentals of spirometry and provide hands-on instruction in small groups with experienced instructors. Students must demonstrate their ability to properly prepare for and administer a spirometry test, verify equipment calibration, and recognize unacceptable maneuvers. NIOSH-approved spirometry refresher courses are also approved for those experienced with spirometry; both types of courses are listed on the NIOSH web page at http://www.cdc.gov/niosh/topics/spirometry/training.html.

Some OSHA standards (e.g., asbestos, benzene) require training for spirometry technicians who are not licensed physicians, and the cotton dust standard specifies that technicians who are not licensed physicians complete a NIOSH-approved course (see 29 CFR 1910.1001, 1910.1028, and 1910.1043). In addition to these regulatory requirements, OSHA recommends that all technicians and other persons conducting occupational spirometry tests obtain certification by completing a NIOSH-approved course and maintain that certification by periodically taking refresher courses.

Since occupational spirometry technicians often perform spirometry tests as only one of many clinical responsibilities, supervisors and directors of spirometry programs should also understand the elements of valid tests and be able to recognize flawed results. Such oversight permits problems to be corrected quickly and tests to be repeated when needed. So that PLHCPs can perform this oversight function, OSHA recommends that supervisors and/or interpreters of test results also complete a NIOSH-approved spirometry course or equivalent training that emphasizes recognition and trouble-shooting of technical errors and the interpretation of spirometry results.

Certificates of successful course completion are issued to individual technicians who have successfully completed a NIOSH-approved course. Institutions or medical practices cannot be "NIOSH-approved" for spirometry testing and the courses are not designed to train medical personnel who subsequently train their staff, unlike some other medical skill training courses. Since each technician who will conduct occupational spirometry tests should complete a NIOSH-approved course, OSHA recommends that program directors identify a limited number of technicians to perform spirometry tests and have them trained, rather than allowing untrained employees to perform the tests. As the designated technicians become more skillful at performing spirometry tests with increasing experience, the program's overall test quality generally will improve.

OSHA recommends that all persons conducting occupational spirometry testing successfully complete an initial NIOSH-approved spirometry course and maintain that certification over time. Some OSHA standards specifically require that health personnel who are not licensed physicians complete a spirometry training course if they test workers covered under those standards.

2.2 EQUIPMENT

2.2.1 SELECTING A SPIROMETER

Types of spirometers. Spirometry tests are performed on volume- and flow-type spirometers (Figures 2 and 3). Volume-type spirometers accumulate air (Figure 2) and directly measure the worker's volume of exhaled air. In contrast, flow-type spirometers (Figure 3) measure the speed of exhaled air and integrate those speeds to obtain volumes of exhaled air. Both types of spirometers can display the volume-time and flow-volume curves shown in Figure 1, and both should meet the spirometer recommendations discussed below and summarized in the text box on OSHA's recommendations for newly-purchased spirometers.

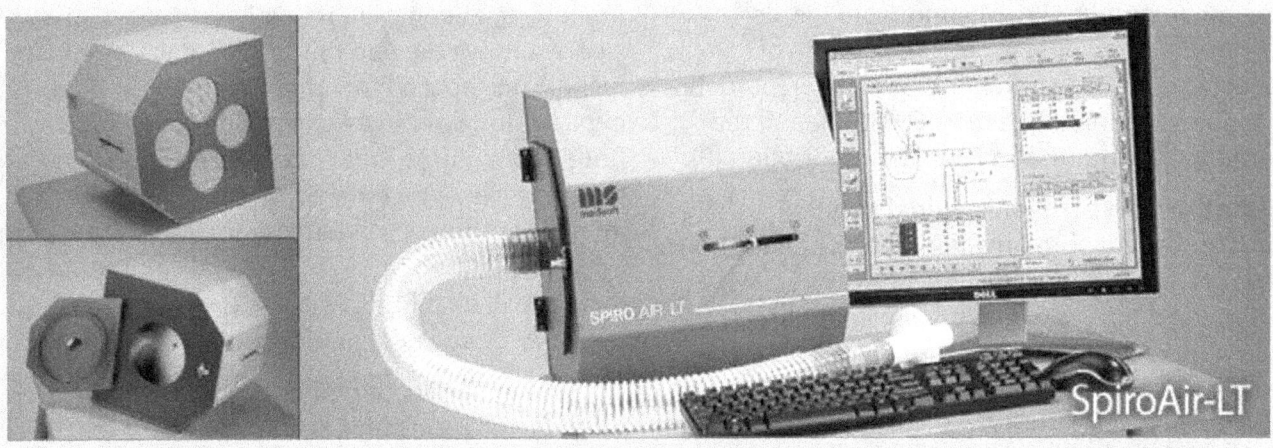

Figure 2. **Example of a volume spirometer with real-time display.**

Image courtesy of Morgan Scientific, Inc. These images are for informational purposes only and do not represent an official OSHA endorsement of the product shown or their manufacturer.

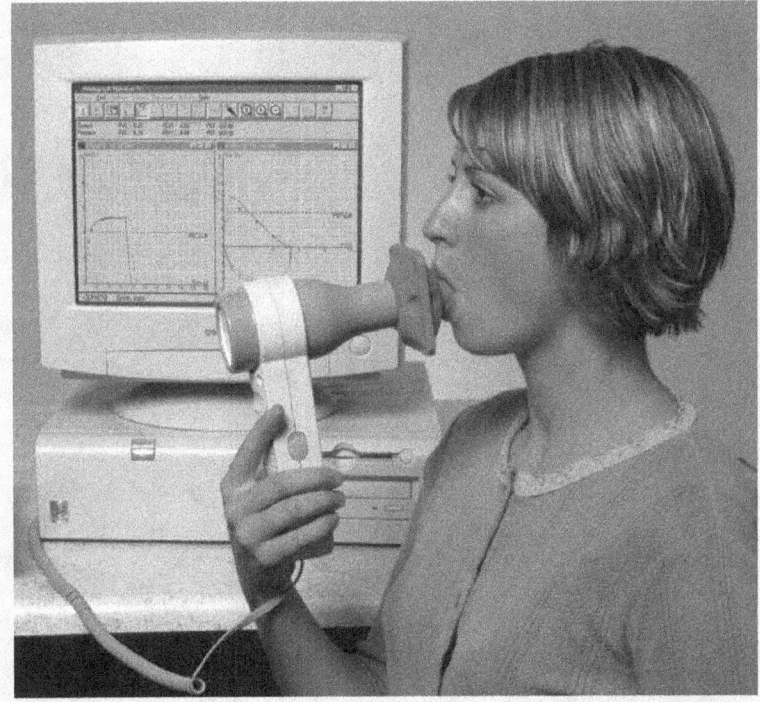

Figure 3. **Example of a flow spirometer sensor with mouthpiece, filter, and real-time display.**

Image courtesy of Vitalograph. This image is for informational purposes only and does not represent an official OSHA endorsement of the products shown or their manufacturer.

Accuracy and Precision. To be useful in occupational health programs, spirometry test results should be accurate, i.e., free from errors. For example, if 3 liters (L) of air are put into a spirometer, the result should be recorded as 3 L. The results should also be precise, or repeatable, e.g., if 3 L of air are put into a spirometer several times, it should be recorded repeatedly as 3 L. Results that are accurate and precise can be compared across different settings and from one time to another (8). Minimum standards for spirometer accuracy, precision, range of measurements, and other operating characteristics have been specified by the ATS/ERS (3) and the International Organization for Standardization (9).

Validation Testing. Independent testing laboratories and some manufacturers perform validation testing to evaluate a prototype spirometer's accuracy and precision under laboratory conditions. Validation testing by independent laboratories is preferred but is not always possible. Before purchasing a spirometer, OSHA recommends that users obtain written verification from the manufacturer that a prototype of that spirometer was tested and met at least the ATS/ERS minimum specifications for accuracy and precision.

However, when the spirometer will be used to evaluate changes in lung function over time, it is also recommended that medical personnel select a spirometer that is even more accurate and precise than the minimum standards (see section 3.2 on Evaluating Results Over Time).

Graphical Displays. Spirometers used for occupational testing should have real-time displays, showing curves while the test is being performed, that are large enough to be viewed easily. By observing real-time displays of both flow-volume and volume-time curves, the technician can judge the worker's effort and provide optimal coaching. Since the flow-volume display emphasizes the beginning of expiration, it helps technicians detect problems early in the maneuver. In contrast, the volume-time display clearly shows the end of the maneuver and helps technicians coach workers to record complete expirations. Spirometers should also include both flow-volume and volume-time curves in their reports of test results to assist PLHCPs in interpreting test results. Reports including adequately sized flow-volume and volume-time graphs will help PLHCPs clearly see problems in the early or late stages of the maneuver.

However, medical personnel should note that manufacturer claims that a spirometer meets ATS/ERS accuracy and precision recommendations may not mean that the display and graph sizes are adequate, since these aspects are not evaluated during validation testing. The recommended minimum sizes for real-time spirometer displays and spirometry report graphs are shown in Figures 4a and 4b.

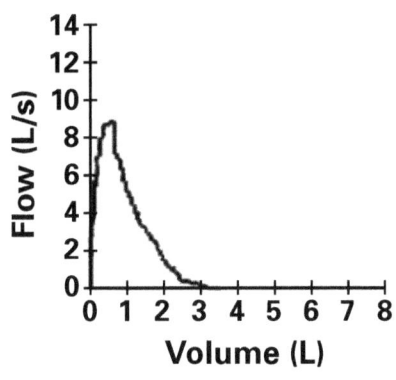

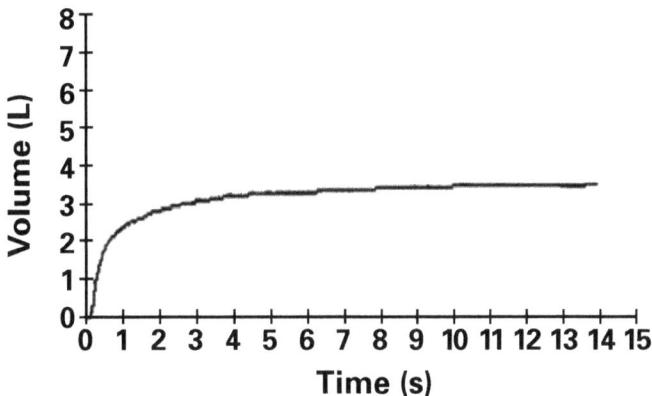

- Volume Scale ≥ 5 mm/L
- Flow Scale ≥ 2.5 mm/L/s
- Time Scale ≥ 5 mm/s

*Complies with ANSI ISO 25672 aspect ratio requirements.

Figure 4a – **ATS/ERS recommended minimum size for real-time spirometer displays during testing.***

Reproduced with permission from ACOEM (5).

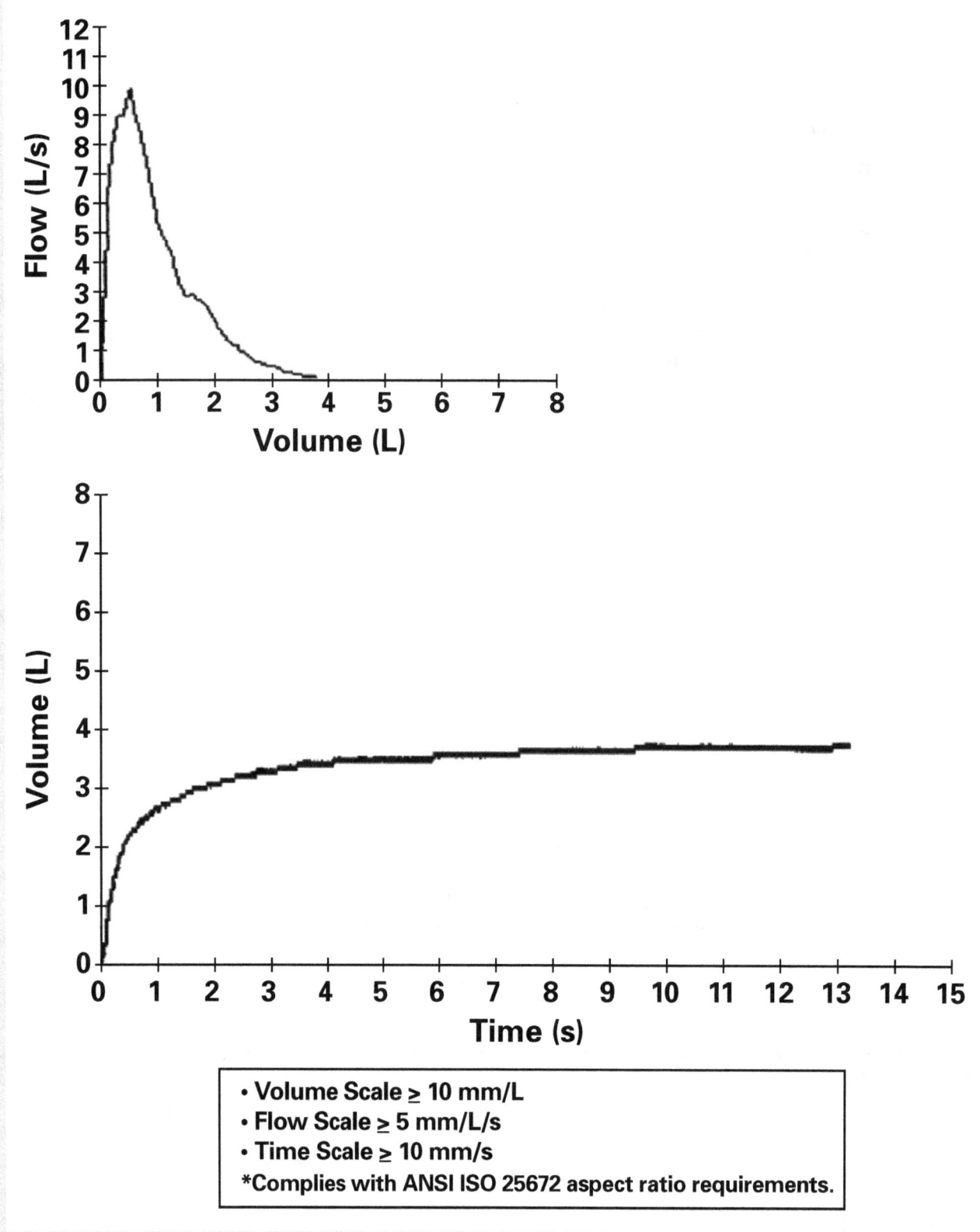

*Figure 4b – **ATS/ERS recommended size for spirometry test report graphic displays.***
Reproduced with permission from ACOEM (5).

Data and Curve Storage and Recall. Other important spirometer aspects relate to information saved from a test session, flexibility of spirometer software in permitting editing of earlier efforts within a test, and choice of output to be included in reports of test results. Poor performance on any of these features can significantly impact the ease with which personnel can conduct occupational spirometry tests and interpret their results.

2.2.2 CHECKING SPIROMETER CALIBRATION

When the spirometer is in use, technicians should verify its accuracy by frequently checking its calibration and performing maintenance procedures at regular intervals. An inaccurate spirometer can produce falsely reduced or elevated worker test results. Such inaccuracies are not always obvious on visual inspection of the test curves. Frequent calibration checks allow for early identification of equipment problems, avoiding weeks or months of reporting incorrect values.

Calibration checks should be performed in the environment in which workers will be tested, and should be conducted:

- At least daily when workers are to be tested;
- Whenever the equipment is changed or relocated; and
- Before the first test and at least every 4 hours on days when large numbers of tests are conducted; this will prevent an undetected problem from invalidating large numbers of test results.

For many models of spirometers, the calibration is checked but cannot be adjusted by the user. If these spirometers become inaccurate and repeatedly fail their calibration checks, and there are no obvious mechanical causes for the inaccuracy, they must be recalibrated by the manufacturer. However, other spirometer models are recalibrated regularly by the technician, who must carefully follow the manufacturer's instructions. After recalibrating such spirometers, technicians should then perform the calibration checks described below. Technicians should use spirometer software programs designed for calibration checks whenever possible.

OSHA recommends that newly purchased spirometers have the following features:

1. Accuracy and precision meet minimum ATS/ERS standards in all cases, and exceed the standards if used to evaluate changes over time in an individual's lung function;
2. Capacity to save and recall all curves and results from up to 8 maneuvers;
3. Ability to electronically save curves and results for simplified future recall and review of test quality and results;
4. Capability to edit and delete previous erroneous curves within a test session;
5. Displays as large as those shown in Figure 4a of both flow-volume and volume-time curves *as the test is being performed* to permit technicians to fully evaluate test quality before deciding whether to save an effort;
6. Automatic calculation and saving of quality control aids, to help with, but not replace, visual evaluation of test quality by well-informed personnel;
7. Display of all data and curves as large as those shown in Figure 4b in the report;
8. Interpretation of largest FVC and FEV_1, even if they occur on different curves;
9. Identification of the reference values (e.g., Hankinson 1999) used in the report;
10. Display of both the predicted values and lower limits of normal (LLN), discussed below, in the report;
11. Display of the FVC and FEV_1 repeatability in the report;
12. A dedicated "calibration check" routine, discussed below, on the spirometer menu; and
13. Display of last calibration check date on each report.

Failure to pass all spirometer checks indicates that workers should not be tested until the cause of failure is identified and corrected, and the spirometer passes all of its calibration checks.

Checks of volume spirometers differ from checks of flow-type spirometers since the goal of the checks is to reveal specific problems unique to each type of equipment.

Volume-type spirometer calibration checks: The first daily check for a volume spirometer is to determine whether it is airtight. Leaks can develop in the hose, the spirometer itself, or connections and seals when spirometers are disassembled for cleaning or when hoses are changed between workers being tested. Small but problematic leaks cannot be detected by inspection alone, so testing for leaks should be conducted daily and when hoses are changed. To test for leaks, inject about 3 L of air into the spirometer and apply a small positive pressure (as recommended by the manufacturer) for one minute while the spirometer outlet (i.e., end of the breathing hose) is blocked. A volume loss of more than 0.03 L/min., i.e., 30 milliliters/minute (ml/min.), indicates a leak that should be corrected before testing workers.

After verifying that there are no leaks, the spirometer's accuracy is checked by injecting 3.00 L of air from a calibration syringe. If the spirometer's recorded volume is within ±3.5% of the injected 3 L, or 2.90–3.10 L, the spirometer is acceptably accurate.

Volume linearity should be checked quarterly. Volume linearity evaluates whether the spirometer is accurate, not just from 0–3 L, as tested daily, but also across its entire volume range. Accuracy in volume linearity is important when workers with large lung volumes are tested. To test for volume linearity, air is manually drawn into the spirometer and its volume is recorded. Then, a 3-L volume of air is injected with a calibration syringe to determine whether the spirometer's recorded volume increases by 3 L.

For example, if 3 L of air from a calibration syringe are injected into a spirometer that already contains 2 L of air, the spirometer's recorded volume should increase to 5 L. If the spirometer already contains 4 L of air, injecting an additional 3 L should increase the spirometer's recorded volume to 7 L. Volume linearity can be checked in three steps, e.g., starting with 0, 2, and 4 L already in the spirometer before using the syringe to inject an additional 3 L of air. Volume linearity can also be checked in more detail, e.g., starting with 0, 1, 2, 3, 4, and 5 L of air in the spirometer and then using a syringe to inject an additional 3 L of air each time. If the spirometer's recorded volume increases by ±3.5% of 3 L, or 2.90–3.10 L in response to each injection, regardless of the starting volume of air in the spirometer, the spirometer is accurate across its entire range and it passes its linearity check.

If a chart drive is used, the speed of the chart drive should also be checked quarterly. To do this, check that the pen takes 10 seconds (s) ± 2% or 9.8–10.2 s to traverse a strip of chart paper that is marked as 10 s in length.

Flow-type spirometer calibration checks: On a daily basis, check the calibration of flow-type spirometers by injecting 3 L of air from a calibration syringe at three different speeds. The syringe should be emptied once in approximately 0.5 s (6 L/s), once in 3 s (1 L/s), and once in 6 s (0.5 L/s). If the spirometer has no time scale, use a clock or watch to gauge the speed of injection. (If needed, count "one-one-thousand, two-one-thousand" etc., while emptying the syringe, to gauge the speed of emptying.) In response to each injection, the spirometer should read within +/- 3.5 percent of 3 L, or 2.90–3.10 L. Failure to record a value in this range at even one of the speeds indicates that the injection should be repeated, and the cause of the incorrect value should be identified and repaired. Often the 6-second injection detects problems with loose connections, aging parts, and sensor problems. Failure at any speed indicates that spirometry testing should not be performed using the spirometer until corrections are made and all speeds are accurate.

If using disposable sensors, a new sensor should be used for each day's calibration check since accuracy of sensors can vary within and between batches. Ideally, the calibration check should be performed with the same sensor that each worker will use, but this is often not possible because of time constraints.

Daily Calibration Checks

Volume Spirometers*:

1. Check that there are no leaks causing an air loss > 0.030 L/min. (30 ml/min.).
2. Inject 3 L air and verify that the recorded value is between 2.90 and 3.10 L.

*Quarterly checks are also needed for volume spirometers – see text for details.

Flow Spirometers:

1. Inject 3 L air at three speeds (taking approximately 0.5 s, 3 s, and 6 s).
2. Verify that the recorded value is between 2.90 and 3.10 L at all three speeds.

Do not conduct worker spirometry tests if the spirometer fails any calibration checks, until the cause of the failure is identified and corrected.

Care of the Calibration Syringe: Store the calibration syringe with the spirometer so that both are in the same environment but out of direct sunlight and away from cold and heat sources. Return the syringe to the manufacturer for recalibration periodically (e.g., every 1–3 years), when the syringe is dropped or damaged, or when its adjustable stops are reset or accidentally moved.

Technicians should leak test the calibration syringe periodically (e.g., monthly) by attempting to empty it with the outlet corked. If a leak is discovered, the syringe should be returned to the manufacturer for repair and recalibration.

2.2.3 AVOIDING SENSOR ERRORS AND ZERO-FLOW ERRORS

Some flow-type spirometer sensors become contaminated or develop zero-flow reference errors during worker tests, producing erroneous and invalid test results. Because these sensor errors occur during spirometry testing, they are not prevented by merely passing a calibration check and often are not identified as errors by the spirometer. To prevent seriously flawed interpretations, users should learn to recognize and delete the flawed curves produced by these errors and develop protocols to prevent and/or to correct the problems if these curves are observed. More information on these errors and how to recognize them is provided below.

Sensor Contamination. Water vapor condensation, secretions, or a worker's fingers can block or contaminate a flow-type spirometer sensor during a test, increasing its resistance. Sensor contamination leads to test results that are falsely *increased* (i.e., larger than actual FEV_1 or FVC), not repeatable, and invalid. Water vapor condensation or secretions may cause FEV_1 and FVC measurements to erroneously increase with each successive maneuver as the sensor becomes increasingly contaminated (Figure 5). This problem may be confused with a learning effect that is observed when a worker inhales more deeply on consecutive maneuvers. However, if the increases in FEV_1 and/or FVC from one maneuver to the next are very large, e.g., > 0.40 L (400 ml), they are unlikely to be caused by a learning effect. If the worker's true lung function is above average, sensor contamination may produce unrealistically high results.

Sensor contamination is not identified by spirometers, so flawed curves should be visually identified and deleted during the test. If a spirometer is vulnerable to this problem, workers should be instructed to keep their fingers away from the sensor outlet and to hold sensors upright (parallel to the floor or pointing to the ceiling) to minimize condensation accumulation. Technicians should frequently check sensors for moisture and mucus accumulation and replace sensors if they become contaminated during a test.

> Technicians should learn to recognize flawed curves resulting from sensor contamination or zero-flow errors and delete such curves. See Figures 5–8 for more details.

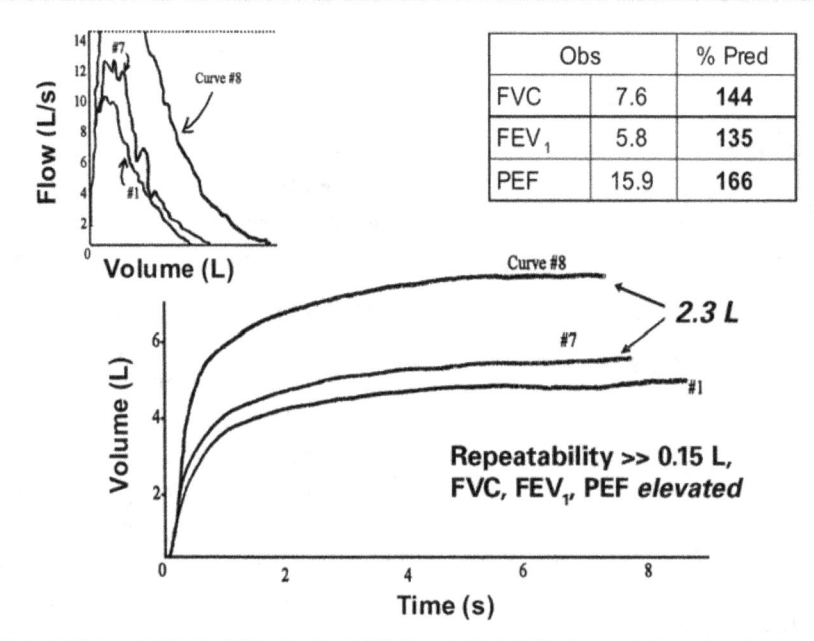

Figure 5. **Error: Sensor Contaminated or Blocked by Condensation, Mucus, or Fingers.**
DELETE THIS TEST. *The last curve (#8) shows the impact of blockage or contamination of the sensor after the 7th maneuver was recorded. The FVC and FEV_1 values are falsely increased on curve #8, exceeding values from the earlier maneuvers (curves #1 and #7) by more than 0.40 L. Technicians must replace the sensor if it becomes contaminated during the test.*

Reprinted with permission from Chest (10).

Zero-Flow Errors. Most flow-type spirometers set a zero-flow reference point before each maneuver, and a few models set the reference point before a complete set of maneuvers. All subsequent flows are measured relative to this reference point. If sensor motion or movements of background air cause slight airflow through the sensor while it is zeroing, the "zero-flow" reference is incorrect and all subsequently measured flows are invalid (Figures 6,7,8).

Zero-flow errors can also be caused by movement of the gravity-sensitive pressure transducer as a worker moves during a test, loose pressure tubing, a degrading sensor, or unstable electronics. Most spirometers do not identify this problem unless it is large, so users should visually identify and delete flawed curves caused by zero-flow errors. Consult Figures 6–8 for information on how to identify these flawed curves. Blocking the sensor during "zeroing" and holding the sensor still during the spirometry test often prevents the problem.

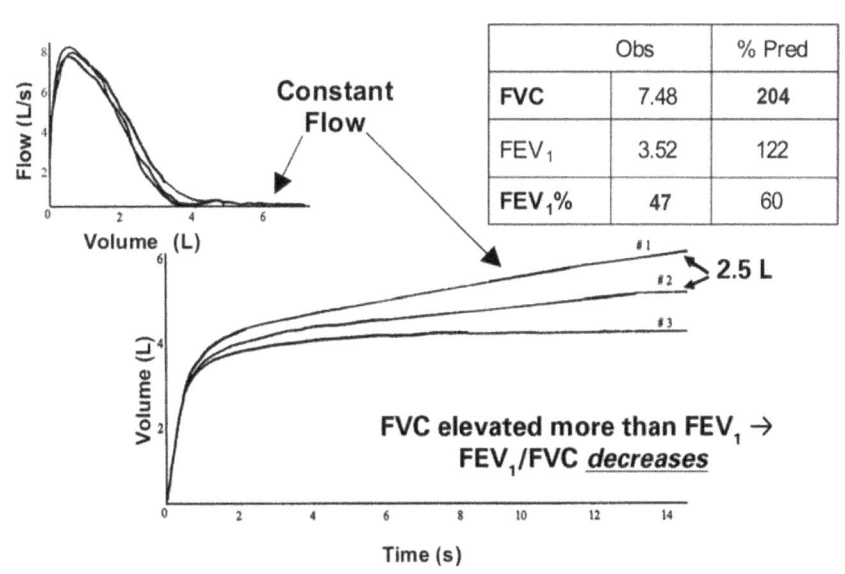

Figure 6. **Error: Inconsistent Zero-Flow Errors Causing Flows to be Over-Recorded.** *DELETE THIS TEST. This spirometer's zero-flow reference point was set at different incorrect levels before the first two maneuvers, causing the volume-time curves (bottom figure) to be splayed apart and extended tails to be drawn to the right on the flow-volume curves (top figure). FVC is increased more than FEV_1, falsely reducing the FEV_1/FVC and probably leading to an erroneous "obstructive impairment" pattern. Block sensor when the spirometer is zeroed and hold sensor still during subject testing to avoid this problem.*

Reprinted with permission from Chest (10).

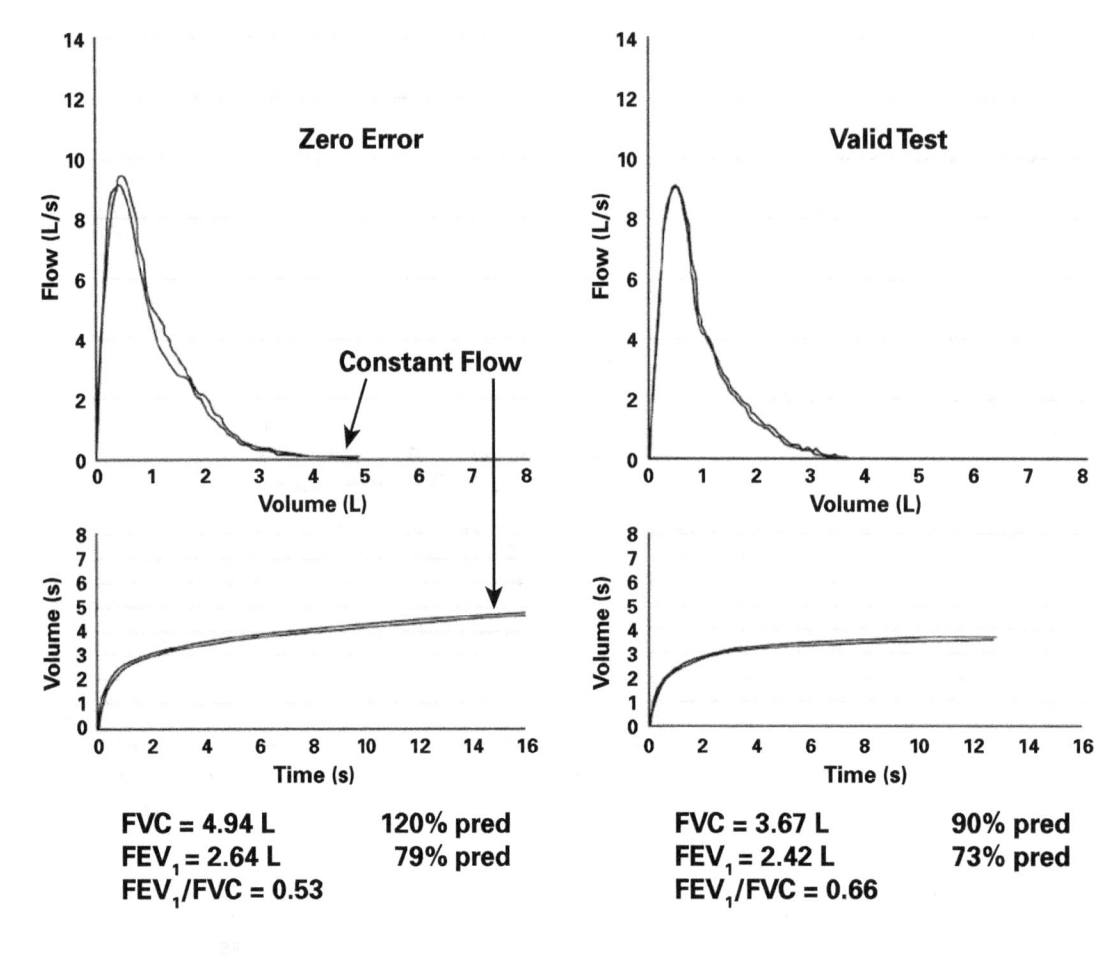

*Figure 7. **Error: Consistent Zero-Flow Error Causing Flows to be Over-Recorded (left).** DELETE THIS TEST. This spirometer's zero-flow reference point was set only once per test, before a complete set of maneuvers. The test on the left shows a zero-flow error, while the test on the right shows valid results; both tests were recorded by the same subject. The zero-flow error on the left produced erroneous but consistent results for all maneuvers, elevating the FVC more than the FEV_1 and falsely reducing the FEV_1/FVC. This zero-flow error may erroneously indicate an "obstructive impairment" pattern. Consistency of the flawed curves on the left may make this error difficult to detect, but technicians should watch out for extended tails that are drawn to the right on the flow-volume curves (top figure), and volume-time curves that climb at a constant rate without reaching a plateau, until the spirometer terminates data collection (bottom figure). Block the sensor when the spirometer is zeroed and hold sensor still during subject testing to avoid this problem.*

Reproduced with permission from ACOEM (5).

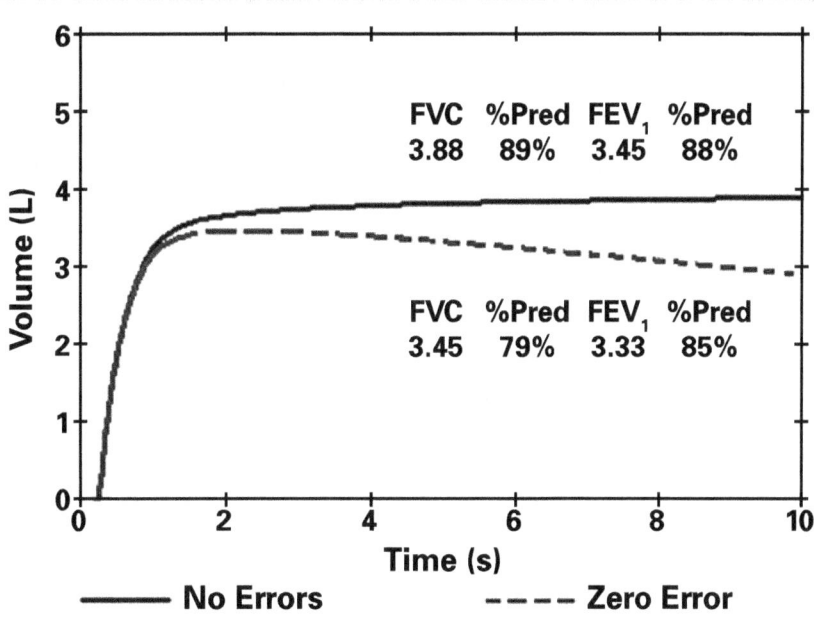

*Figure 8. **Error: Zero-Flow Error Causing Flows to be Under-Recorded.** FVC is much more reduced than FEV_1, falsely increasing the FEV_1/FVC and possibly masking true airways obstruction. Block the sensor when the spirometer is zeroed and hold sensor still during subject testing to avoid this problem.*

Reprinted with permission from ACOEM (5).

2.2.4 INFECTION CONTROL

There is a potential risk for transmission of infection through spirometry equipment. Technicians should follow manufacturer's recommendations for spirometer cleaning and maintenance. NIOSH (8) recommends that technicians:

1. Wash hands before and after administering a spirometry test;
2. Instruct workers to attach, remove and discard the disposable mouthpiece themselves;
3. Use disposable or sterilized noseclips;
4. Do not test workers who have active respiratory infections (e.g., a cold or the flu);
5. Use a clean breathing tube for each worker tested with a volume spirometer;
6. Consider using disposable spirometry filters for volume spirometers;
7. Do not reuse flow sensors designed for single patient use for flow spirometers;
8. Follow the spirometer manufacturer's recommendations for cleaning and disinfecting the equipment;
9. Disinfect hard surfaces by wiping them with antimicrobial cleaners; and
10. Follow mandates from your institution and your state health department on infection control in healthcare settings.

2.3 CONDUCTING SPIROMETRY TESTS

2.3.1 PREPARING THE WORKER FOR TESTING

Before conducting spirometry testing, the technician should interview the worker, review medical records, and possibly consult with the PLHCP to identify health conditions that may prevent the worker from safely performing maximal efforts in a spirometry test. The ATS/ERS (2) suggests not performing spirometry when the following are present:

- Myocardial infarction within the past month;
- Chest/abdominal pain;
- Oral/facial pain that is aggravated by the mouthpiece;
- Stress incontinence; or
- Dementia/confusion.

In addition, other groups (8, 16) recommend postponing spirometry for:

- One hour after smoking, using a bronchodilator, or eating a heavy meal;
- Three days after recovering from an illness that lasted three weeks or less;
- Three weeks after a severe respiratory illness or ear infection; and
- Six or more weeks after eye, ear, chest, or abdominal surgery, unless a surgeon provides a release statement.

After determining that the worker can be tested:

- Record the worker's age and race/ethnicity, based on the worker's self-report;
- Measure height (and weight) without shoes, since self-reported height and weight may be inaccurate;
- Loosen tight clothing, such as neckties, back braces, protective vests, and some belts, bras or girdles, if they will restrict maximal breathing;
- Remove dentures only if loose;
- Check for dental work or piercings that may interfere with mouthpiece placement or proper lip seal; and
- Apply disposable noseclips.

Recording the worker's age and race/ethnicity, as well as measuring exact height, is important because a worker's normal range of lung function is determined by these factors. Weight does not affect the normal range but should be considered when interpreting results. Increased weight around the midsection can restrict the worker's ability to take a full breath, thereby reducing lung function in the absence of lung disease.

Disposable noseclips are recommended to prevent extra inhalations through the nose at the end of the maneuver. If noseclips do not fit properly, have the worker pinch his/her nostrils closed while performing each maneuver.

2.3.2 TEST POSTURE

Recently, ACOEM (5) recommended that workers stand while performing spirometry tests. NIOSH (8) also recommends that workers stand for their spirometry tests. In 2005, the ATS/ERS (3) recommended that patients sit during pulmonary function testing for safety reasons. OSHA recommends that workers stand during spirometry testing unless they cannot do so because of a safety or health concern such as a history of fainting or an illness. OSHA's recommendation is based on the following reasons:

- Most workers are healthy enough to stand during testing;
- Slightly larger lung volumes are recorded by many workers when standing; and
- Workers who are obese or have extra weight at the midsection often take deeper breaths and exhale larger volumes when standing.

If the worker stands for the test, take the following safety precautions:

- Place a sturdy chair without wheels behind the worker;
- Watch the worker during testing for signs of light-headedness;
- Place a hand on the worker's arm or back if needed to steady them; and
- Stop the test if any signs of distress are observed.

If the worker experiences light-headedness, fainting, or any other signs of distress during testing, the problem should be documented and future testing of the worker should be conducted in the seated posture.

Under all circumstances:

- The worker should stand or sit upright, with their chin slightly elevated, and with their tongue beneath and lips tightly sealed around the mouthpiece; and
- The testing posture should be documented and future spirometry tests should be conducted in the same standing or sitting position.

Figure 9 shows the proper posture during testing.

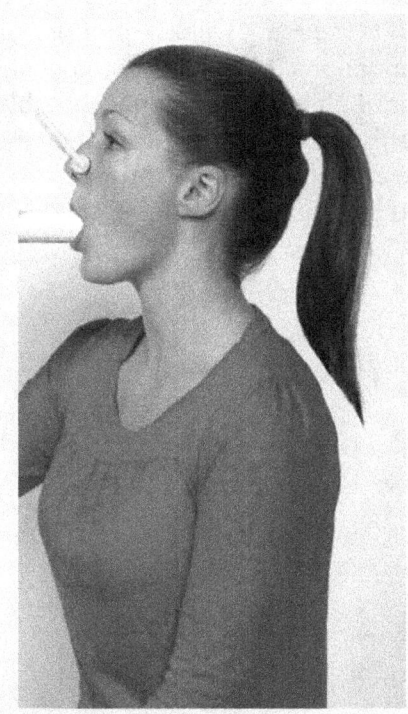

Figure 9. **Proper Posture During Spirometry.**

Image courtesy of Vitalograph. This image is for informational purposes only and does not represent an official OSHA endorsement of the company providing this image.

2.3.3 PERFORMING THE TEST

To obtain accurate spirometry test results, the worker should successfully perform the three distinct steps of the forced expiratory maneuver:

1. Inhale *maximally* at the start of the test;
2. Blast the air out as hard and as fast as possible; and
3. Continue to exhale one breath until it is fully recorded.

Performing a Forced Expiratory Maneuver

The technician *explains, demonstrates,* and actively *coaches* the worker. To obtain meaningful results, the technician should:

1. **Explain** how to perform the test:
   - Explain the purpose of the test – "to see how much air your lungs can hold and how hard and fast you can blast it out;"
   - Take the deepest possible breath to fill your lungs;
   - Place the mouthpiece on top of the tongue and between the teeth;
   - Seal lips tightly around the mouthpiece, making sure not to purse the lips behind the mouthpiece;
   - Slightly elevate the chin and keep the tongue out of the way of the mouthpiece;
   - Blast, without hesitating, into the mouthpiece as hard, fast, and completely as possible; and
   - Keep blowing as long as you can, or until you are told to stop.

2. **Demonstrate** how to use the mouthpiece: fill the lungs, blast out immediately, and keep exhaling as long as possible. The entire maneuver should be demonstrated, exaggerating each step if helpful, even if the worker has performed the test previously.

3. **Coach** the worker to perform the maneuver: "Fill your lungs and when you're ready, blast the air out, push, keep going, keep going" until the end of test. (8)

The technician should observe that the worker understood the instructions and performed the maneuver with a maximum inspiration, a good start, a smooth continuous exhalation, and maximal effort. The worker can relax for as long as needed after each maneuver, while the technician checks the acceptability of the completed effort. If the curve was not acceptable (described below), the technician should identify (and perhaps demonstrate) specific errors and instruct the worker on how to correct the problems before proceeding with the next effort.

2.3.4 ELEMENTS OF A VALID TEST

The goal of spirometry testing is to obtain accurate measurements of lung function. A "valid" test includes at least three technically "acceptable" maneuvers, described in detail below. Once three acceptable curves are recorded, consistency, i.e., "repeatability," of results is evaluated. When the worker records three acceptable curves with repeatable results, the test is "valid" and can be concluded.

Up to eight efforts can be attempted to record a valid test, unless the worker cannot or should not continue (3). Workers should stop exhaling any time they cannot continue, and they should not perform multiple exhalations lasting longer than 15 seconds. If three acceptable results have not been recorded within five attempts, check that the worker is able to proceed since some individuals with obstructive airways disease may experience too much discomfort to continue.

> Achieving three acceptable curves with repeatable results is a **testing goal**, achievable by most healthy workers, and every effort should be made to reach this goal. However, failure to meet this goal should not necessarily prevent reporting of results, because some workers are not capable of recording valid tests. Records of such maneuvers should be retained since tests that do not meet these criteria can often be interpreted, but the fact that a valid test was not recorded should be noted.

Acceptability

A curve is considered acceptable when the worker performs all aspects of the forced expiratory maneuver correctly. Acceptable spirometry curves display maximal inhalations, hard initial blasts (free of hesitation and cough in the first second), complete exhalations, and maximal effort throughout the maneuver. Figures 10 and 16 below show acceptable curves for forced expirations, and Figures 11–15 and 17 show curves with common problems: incomplete inhalations, hesitations, coughs in the first second, weak expiratory push, and early terminations. Medical personnel should learn to recognize the shapes of unacceptable curves since spirometer quality prompts may be incomplete and are not a substitute for understanding by medical personnel (11).

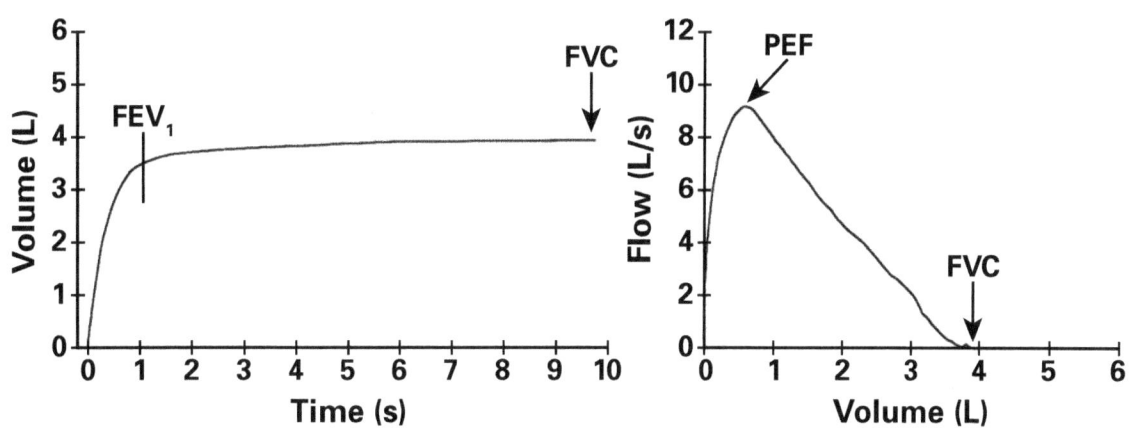

*Figure 10. **Acceptable Test**. As the worker blasts the air out during a forced expiratory maneuver, the volume-time curve (left) shows an initial rapid increase in recorded exhaled volume. The volume then continues to increase slowly until the exhalation is complete and a flat FVC plateau is drawn. The flow-volume curve (right), drawn during the same forced expiration, shows the maximal speed of exhaled air that is achieved immediately, indicated by "PEF," i.e., Peak Expiratory Flow, and the subsequent slowing of expiratory speed as the lungs empty.*

Reproduced with permission from ACOEM (5).

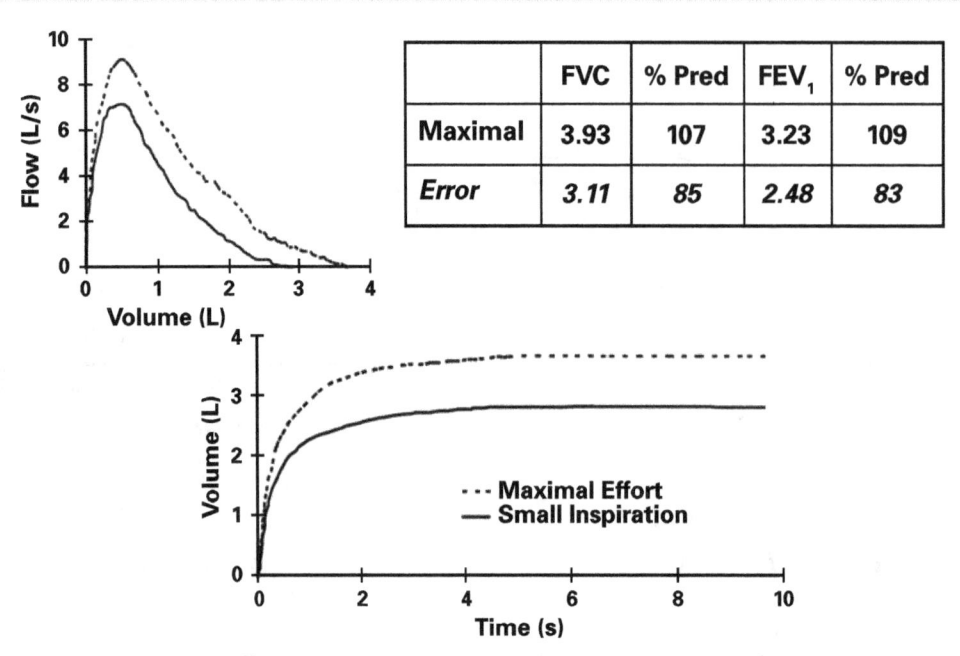

Figure 11. **Error: Incomplete Inspiration (solid curves)**. The solid volume-time curve (bottom figure) resulted from a worker failing to inhale maximally before the forced expiration. The solid curve is considerably lower than the dashed curve that was drawn when the worker inhaled maximally before the forced exhalation. An incomplete inspiration can give the appearance of reduced FEV_1 and FVC, and may cause false spirometer interpretations of "restrictive impairment." Coach the worker: "Fill your lungs."

Reproduced with permission from ACOEM (5).

Curves with initial hesitation or cough are frequently labeled as errors but not deleted by spirometers; *technicians should delete these curves,* even when not prompted by the spirometer to do so. However, coughing toward the end of the maneuver does not affect test results, and the curves can be saved.

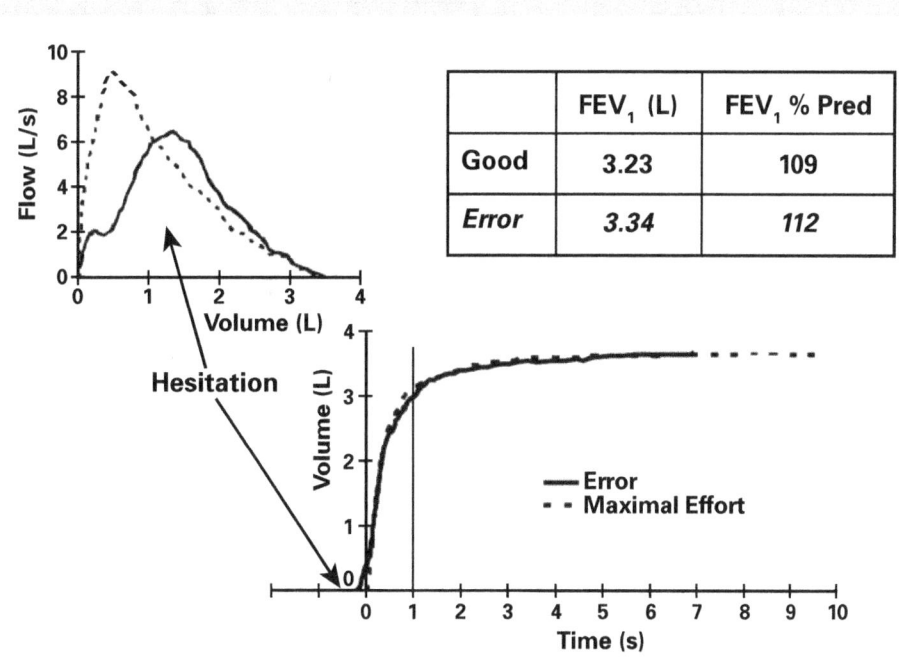

Figure 12. **Error: Excessive Hesitation (solid curves).** *DELETE THIS TEST. Because the worker's initial blast is delayed, the peak of the flow-volume curve (top figure) is displaced to the right, and a gradually climbing tail is seen at the start of the volume-time curve (bottom figure). Coach the worker: "Blast out as soon as you are ready."*

Reproduced with permission from ACOEM (5).

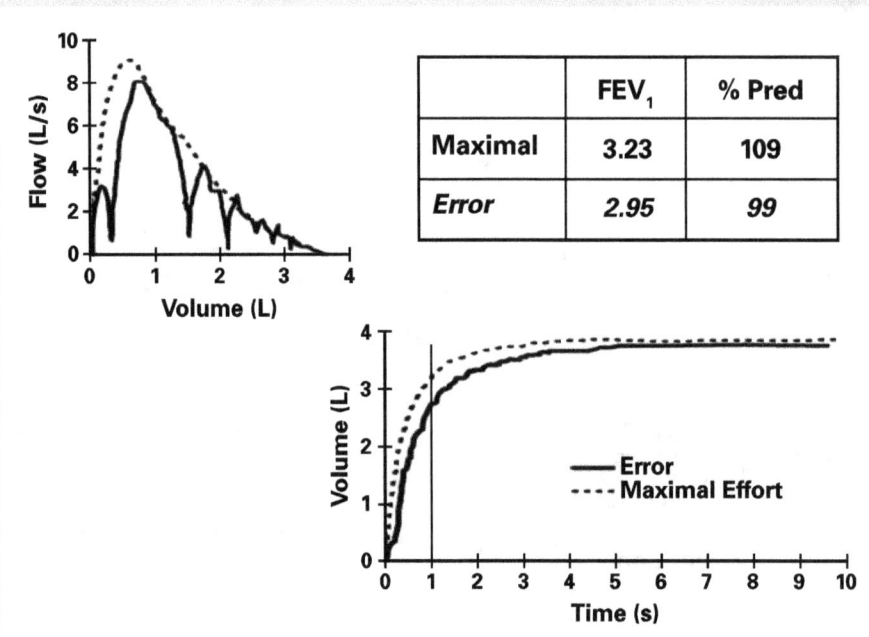

Figure 13. **Error: Cough in 1st Second (solid curves)**. DELETE THIS TEST. Because cough in the first second repeatedly interrupts the airflow early in the expiration, the flow-volume curve (top figure) clearly shows steep changes (interruptions) in the flow rate, while the volume-time curve (bottom figure) shows only subtle steps in the first second. A drink of water sometimes solves this problem.

Reproduced with permission from ACOEM (5).

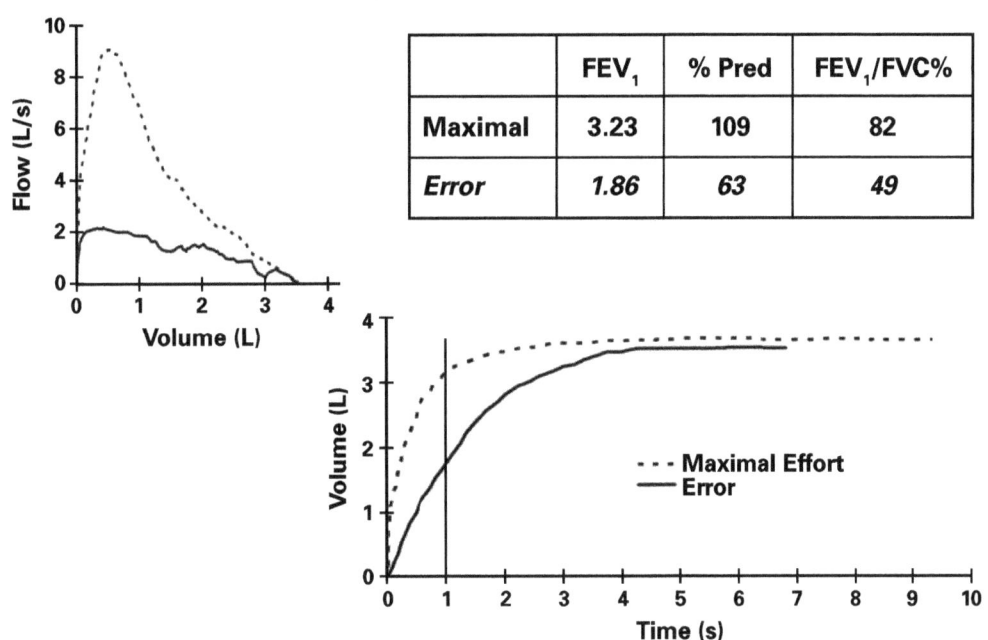

*Figure 14. **Error: No Blast (solid curves)**. This worker failed to blast out initially, so the expiratory speed was never rapid. The flow-volume curve (top figure) has no sharp peak, and the volume-time curve (bottom figure) shows a slanted start of expiration. Such a weak push reduces the FEV_1 and FEV_1/FVC, and may be caused by the worker trying to "save" air so that they can exhale for many seconds. This error causes false spirometer interpretations of "obstructive impairment." Coach "Blast out hard and fast" to solve this problem.*

Reproduced with permission from ACOEM (5).

An acceptable end-of-test is recorded when a one-second FVC plateau is reached by a worker who tries to exhale for 6 or more seconds. Figure 15 shows a test with early termination: no plateau is reached and the FVC is under-recorded, causing the FEV_1/FVC to be incorrectly *elevated*. Coaching should emphasize complete exhalations for the remaining efforts.

In contrast, if a healthy worker with a small lung volume tries to exhale for 6 seconds but reaches the FVC plateau before 6 seconds have elapsed (Figure 16), the test is valid, though many spirometers will erroneously label it as "unacceptable." Normal young workers often complete their expirations in less than 6 seconds.

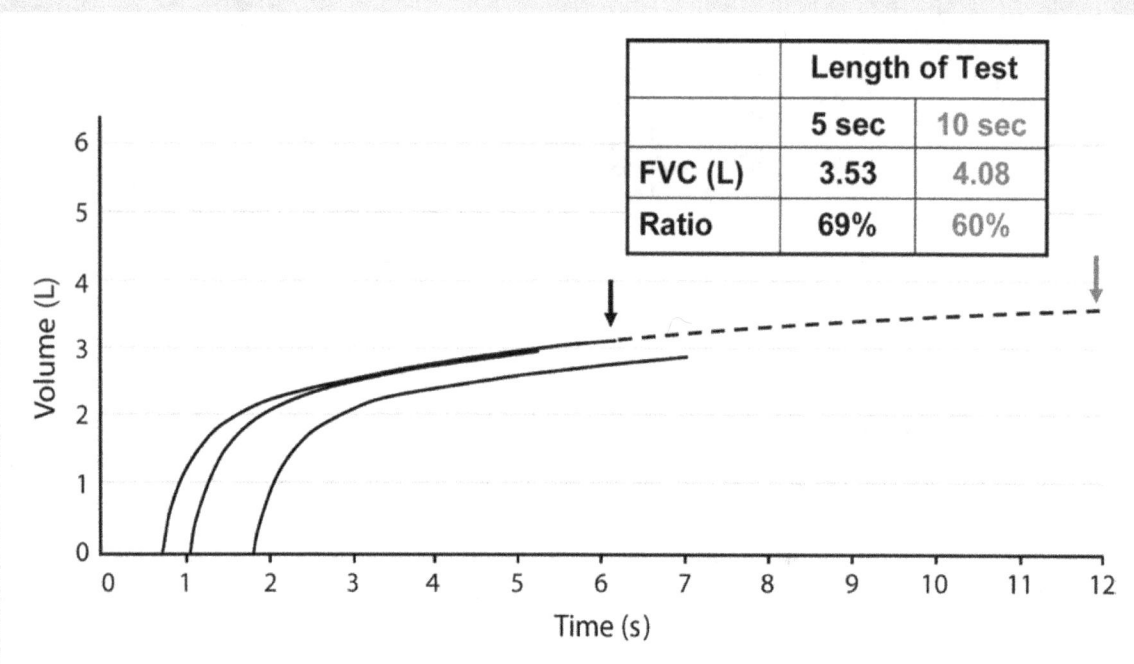

Figure 15. **Error: Early Termination (solid curves).** *When an expiration stops before the volume-time curve flattens into a 1-second plateau, the FVC may not be fully recorded. The solid lines show expirations for a subject with airways obstruction who terminated the exhalations early. Such incomplete recordings falsely* increase *the FEV_1/FVC and may cause the spirometer interpretation to be "normal" even when airways obstruction is present.*

The dashed line shows the increase in FVC that would have occurred with only 5 more seconds of expiration for this subject who cannot reach a plateau within the time shown. The resulting higher FVC and the lower but more accurate FEV_1/FVC *would trigger a correct interpretation of "airways obstruction." (Note: though not shown here, subjects should try to exhale to a 1-second plateau when possible. However, multiple curves longer than 15 seconds should not be recorded.) Coach "Keep blowing until I tell you to stop."*

Reproduced with permission from ACOEM (5).

25 yr 62" WF	Observed	%Pred
FVC	3.76 L	107%
FEV_1	3.30	112%
FEV_1/FVC	88%	105%
Time (FET)	4.5 s	–

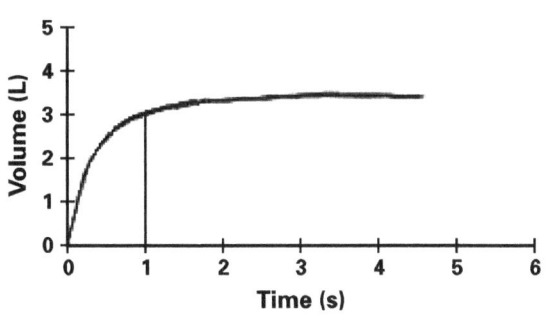
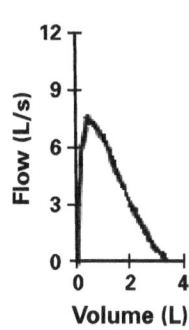

Figure 16. **Acceptable Test with FVC Plateau in < 6 seconds.** *Because the subject tried to exhale for 6 seconds and a 1-second FVC plateau was recorded, the test is acceptable (3). Spirometer error messages about "early termination" or "unacceptable test" should be ignored.*

Reproduced with permission from ACOEM (5).

Curves indicating extra inhalations through the nose at the end of the maneuver (Figure 17) should be deleted, even though they are not labeled as errors by most spirometers. If the worker uses noseclips or pinches his/her nose during expiration, this problem will be avoided.

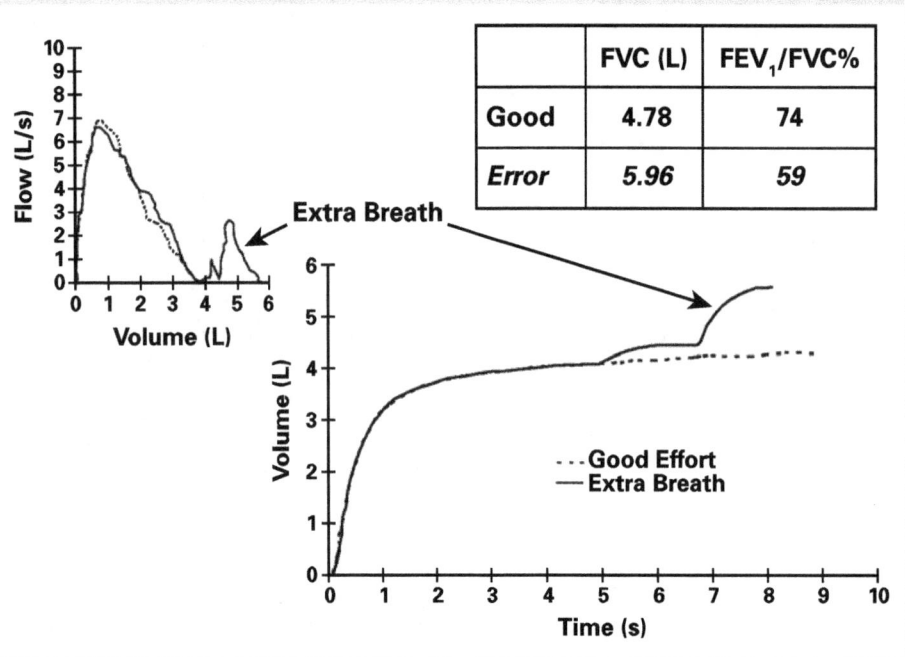

Figure 17. **Error: Extra Breath Through the Nose at End of Test (solid curves). DELETE THIS TEST.** At the end of the forced expiration, this worker inhaled additional air through the nose and quickly exhaled it into the spirometer mouthpiece. The flow-volume curve (top figure) shows multiple maneuvers and the volume-time curve (bottom figure) shows additional expirations in increasing steps at the end of the test. This error erroneously elevates the FVC, greatly reduces the FEV_1/FVC, and causes a false spirometer interpretation of "airways obstruction." Solution: have the worker wear nose clips.

Reproduced with permission from ACOEM (5).

- Some spirometry errors falsely elevate FVC and/or FEV_1: hesitations (Figure 12), extra inhalations (Figure 17), contaminated sensors (Figure 5), and over-recorded flows caused by zero flow errors (Figures 6 and 7). It is especially important to delete these errors because spirometers save the largest test results for interpretation.
- Other errors, such as incomplete inhalations (Figure 11), coughs in the first second of exhalation (Figure 13), and weak expiratory pushes (Figure 14), often falsely reduce FVC and/or FEV_1. Spirometers usually discard such falsely low values when good coaching leads to higher, more accurate results on subsequent maneuvers.
- Interpretation of falsely elevated or reduced results may indicate incorrectly that impairment exists when a worker is normal, or that a worker is normal when impairment in fact exists.

Repeatability

Three acceptable curves in a well-performed test usually have repeatable shapes and consistent results among the maneuvers. Evaluation of the consistency or "repeatability" of the measurements is the final step in determining whether a test is valid and complete. Values for FVC and FEV_1 are considered repeatable when the largest FVC minus the second largest FVC and the largest FEV_1 minus the second largest FEV_1, taken from acceptable curves, are both 0.15 L (150 ml) or less. Repeatability was formerly called "reproducibility" and many spirometers label it as "variability."

Lack of repeatability is often caused by failing to inhale maximally before each maneuver, and coaching should focus on correcting errors by improving inhalations (Figure 11), expiratory blasts (Figure 14), or completeness of the expirations (Figure 15). However, when FVC or FEV_1 repeatability is *very* poor, e.g., >0.40 L (400 ml), it may indicate sensor contamination or zero-flow errors (See Figures 5–8).

Repeatable results can be recorded by most healthy workers when they consistently exert a maximal effort for each maneuver attempted, and every effort should be made to record a valid test. However, workers with airways obstruction sometimes have difficulty achieving repeatability, and as a result, non-repeatable test results should not be excluded from interpretation. Failure to achieve repeatability should be documented and taken into account during interpretation of results.

Results are "repeatable" when the largest FVC minus the second largest FVC and the largest FEV_1 minus the second largest FEV_1, taken from acceptable curves, are both 0.15 L (150 ml) or less.

2.3.5 MEASUREMENTS TO BE REPORTED

As indicated above, spirometry tests measure the maximum exhaled volume (FVC) and speed (FEV_1) that a worker can achieve during a forced expiratory maneuver. Therefore, the largest FVC and FEV_1 values from acceptable efforts are reported, even *if they come from different curves* (3, 5). The FEV_1/FVC is calculated using these two maximal values. Users may need to change their default spirometer configurations to permit the reporting and interpretation of the highest FVC and highest FEV_1 values when they are derived from different curves.

When results for the FEV_1 and FEV_1/FVC are within the normal range, ATS/ERS (4) and ACOEM (5) generally recommend against evaluating Forced Expiratory Flow (FEF) rates, i.e., the instantaneous changes in expiratory flow measured during a forced expiration. But if reported, such flow rates should be drawn from the one overall "best" curve with the highest sum of FEV_1 + FVC. However, for the maximal flow achieved during the forced expiration, i.e., the Peak Expiratory Flow (PEF), the highest value from all acceptable curves should be reported.

Spirometry test reports should present results and volume-time and flow-volume curves from all acceptable maneuvers to permit evaluation of technical quality. In addition, test posture, worker effort and cooperation, date of last spirometer calibration check or calibration, and technician identification (ID) should be recorded on the test report.

3.0 INTERPRETING TEST RESULTS

Before interpreting test results, the PLHCP should evaluate the test's technical quality and determine whether a valid test with acceptable and repeatable results was recorded, as described above. The ATS/ERS cautions that "omitting the quality review and relying only on numerical results for clinical decision making is a common mistake, which is more easily made by those who are dependent upon computer interpretations." (4)

Valid worker results are compared to (1) the normal range expected for a person with the worker's characteristics (gender, age, height, and race/ethnicity), and/or (2) the worker's previous test results. In both cases, worker results are examined to determine whether the measured volume and speed of exhaled air are significantly smaller or slower than expected. Such findings can serve as the basis for decisions about worker respiratory health or the need for medical referrals, as well as actions to be taken in prevention and early intervention programs.

> When interpreting spirometry results, medical personnel should evaluate the technical quality of the test and not rely solely on numerical results and computer interpretations.

3.1 COMPARING WORKER RESULTS WITH THE NORMAL RANGE (REFERENCE VALUES)

Once valid test results have been obtained, correct interpretation of worker respiratory health depends on two factors: (1) selecting and consistently using appropriate reference values to define the normal range for FVC, FEV_1, and FEV_1/FVC; and (2) following an appropriate algorithm to categorize the worker's spirometry results as normal or abnormal.

3.1.1 SELECTING REFERENCE VALUES

The measured FEV_1/FVC, FVC, and FEV_1 values from a worker's valid test are compared with normal ranges specific for the worker's age, measured standing height, gender, and race/ethnicity. Reference values specify both the average "predicted" value and the 5th percentile lower limit of the normal range (LLN). The LLN is defined so that 95 percent of a "normal" nonsmoking population will have values above the LLN and only 5 percent of a "normal" population will have values below the LLN. Comparison of the worker's measured values with reference values will determine whether the worker's lung function is considered to be normal or abnormal.

Reference values that define normal ranges for spirometry measurements are generated by research studies that conduct spirometry tests on large groups of healthy people. The most widely endorsed reference values for use in the U.S. are based on data collected by the National Health and Nutrition Examination Survey III (NHANES III) and published in 1999 by Hankinson. NHANES III studied a diverse U.S. population: spirometry tests were conducted on 8 to 80-year-old male and female non-smoking Caucasians, African-Americans, and Mexican-Americans living in various locations across the United States. The NHANES III study also maintained strict quality control procedures to guarantee that accurate spirometry results of high technical quality were recorded. (12)

Because the NHANES III (Hankinson) reference values were developed from diverse populations using strict quality control, OSHA recommends using those values to interpret occupational spirometry results, unless a specific standard requires a different reference group. For example, the OSHA Cotton Dust standard (29 CFR 1910.1043) mandates use of the Knudson 1976 reference values (13) presented in Appendix C to that standard. However, the Knudson 1976 reference values should not be used except when mandated by that standard. Most new spirometers include the NHANES III (Hankinson) reference values as a configuration option, and this option should be selected. If older spirometers are used for general occupational spirometry testing, OSHA recommends using the reference value calculator at http://cdc.gov/niosh/topics/spirometry/RefCalculator.html or tables of reference values to obtain the NHANES III-based predicted values and LLNs for the worker being tested. The NHANES III reference values are included in Appendix A of this guidance document. PLHCPs who interpret spirometry test results should verify that the source of reference values used to evaluate worker pulmonary function is identified in the spirometry report.

All of a worker's spirometry test results should be evaluated relative to a single set of reference values, regardless of which reference set is selected. However, some spirometers construct composite reference values that combine results from different reference sets, which often vary with respect to measurement techniques, equipment used, and subjects who were studied. Using data from composite reference sets can result in inaccurate characterization of the normal range and, therefore, "composite" normal values should not be used.

> OSHA recommends that spirometry results for workers in the United States be compared with NHANES III (Hankinson 1999) reference values unless an OSHA standard requires that a different reference set be used.

3.1.2 RACE ADJUSTMENT

As noted earlier, the NHANES III reference values provide accurate FVC, FEV_1, and FEV_1/FVC predicted values and LLNs for three broad racial/ethnic groups within the U.S.: Caucasians, African-Americans, and Mexican-Americans. All designations of race or ethnicity are based on self-report, and workers, including bi- or multiracial individuals, should choose the racial/ethnic group that characterizes them best. Diversity exists within each of the NHANES III racial/ethnic groups, but current recommendations are to use the NHANES III reference value set which is closest to the worker's characteristics. Thus the NHANES III Mexican-American reference values are also used for non-Mexican-American Hispanic workers. Because specific reference values are not provided for Asian-American workers, Caucasian reference values for FVC and FEV_1 should be multiplied by an adjustment factor to obtain normal ranges for Asian-Americans. Based on current research (5, 14), OSHA recommends multiplying the Caucasian predicted values and LLNs for FVC and FEV_1 by 0.88 to adjust those values for Asian workers. Since the FEV_1/FVC is relatively unaffected by race, the Caucasian reference values for the FEV_1/FVC are *not* adjusted for differences in race/ethnicity for Asian workers. Other racial/ethnic groups, such as Native American Indians, have lung function that is similar to Caucasians' and no adjustment of the Caucasian reference values is necessary for such workers (8).

3.1.3 APPLYING THE INTERPRETATION ALGORITHM

Spirometry interpretations should specify whether the worker's lung function is in the normal range, or shows an obstructive, restrictive, or mixed impairment pattern. Merely stating which values are normal or low, without concluding if there is an impairment pattern, is not helpful (4).

OSHA recommends following the algorithm pictured in Figure 18 below at page 30 to interpret lung function. This general approach has previously been recommended by ACOEM (5), ATS/ERS (4), and NIOSH (8). Figure 18 lists three steps to be followed in interpreting spirometry test results: first, evaluate the validity of the test results, second, assess whether expiratory airflow is slowed (obstructive impairment), and finally, consider whether expired lung volumes might be reduced (restrictive impairment). It is important to follow the steps in the order specified to minimize false positive findings when interpreting spirometry test results. All three steps must be evaluated for every set of test results.

The algorithm shown in Figure 18 is used to classify the worker as having:

- Obstructive impairment (also called airways obstruction);
- Possible restrictive impairment;
- Possible mixed impairment (both obstructive and possible restrictive impairments); or
- Normal spirometry results (no obstructive or restrictive impairment).

Each of these classifications is described below, following the sequence in Figure 18.

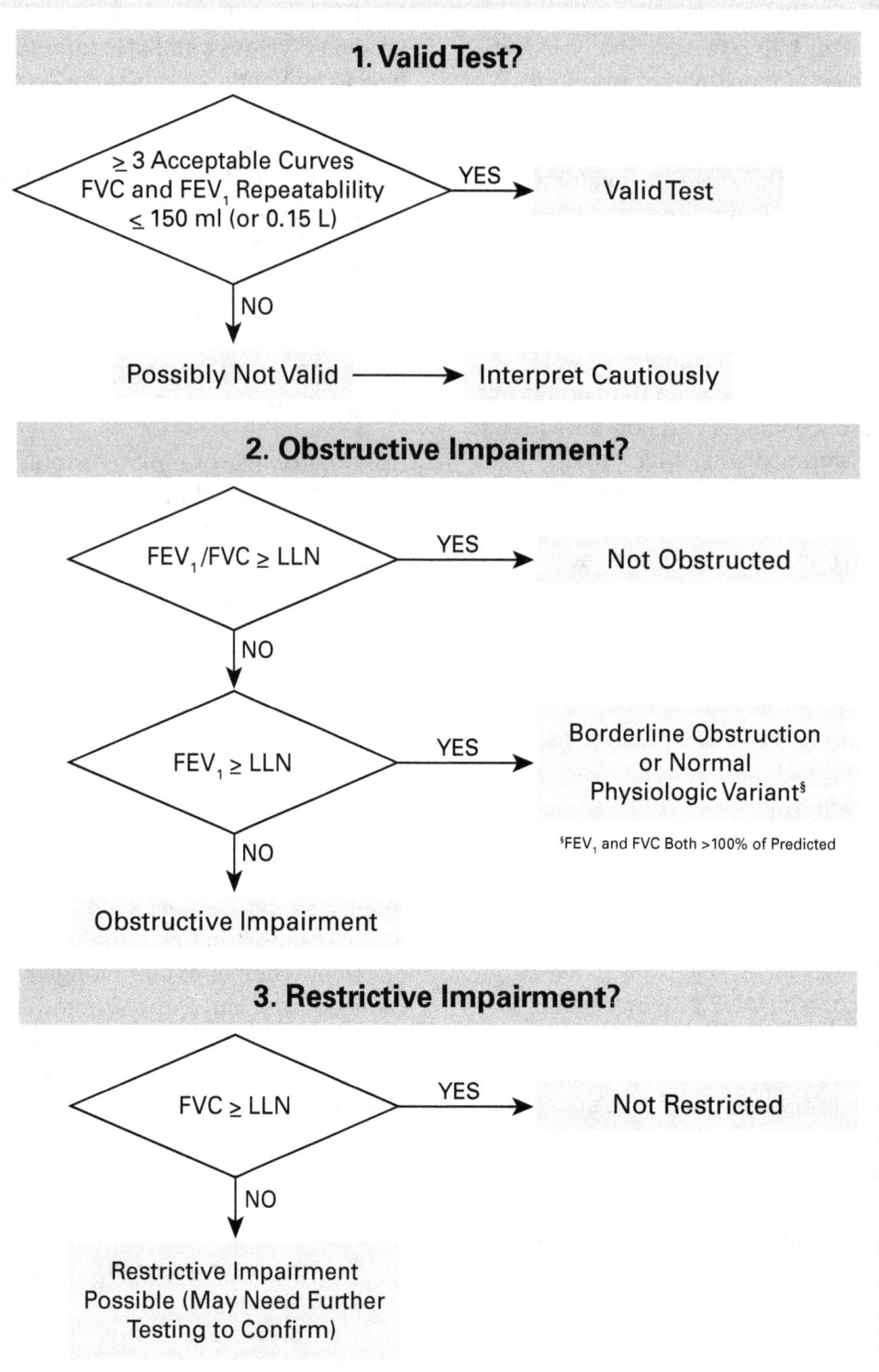

Figure 18. *ACOEM Spirometry Algorithm.*

Adapted from ACOEM (5).

Obstructive Impairment
Step 2 (Figure 18) shows that when a worker's FEV_1/FVC and FEV_1 are both < LLN, *airways obstruction* is present. Workers with obstructive lung diseases, such as Chronic Obstructive Pulmonary Disease (COPD) or chronic asthma often have an abnormally low FEV_1/FVC and a low FEV_1.

When FEV_1/FVC is < LLN, but FEV_1 is ≥ LLN, the worker may exhibit *borderline obstruction or normal physiologic variant. Borderline obstruction* is likely when the FEV_1 is below average, i.e., < 100 percent of predicted FEV_1. The complete clinical picture and exposure history should be considered in such workers and they should be retested at a later date. However, when both the FEV_1 and FVC are above average, i.e., > 100 percent of predicted FEV_1 and FVC, the possibility of a *normal physiologic variant* rather than airways obstruction should be considered. This pattern is not uncommon in physically fit non-smokers such as athletes, emergency responders, firefighters, and police. However, if workers with this pattern are exposed to respiratory hazards known to cause airways obstruction, the possibility of true airways obstruction should be considered.

Restrictive Impairment
Step 3 (Figure 18) shows that when FVC is < LLN, *restrictive impairment* may be present. Further pulmonary function tests to evaluate lung volumes may be required to confirm a restrictive impairment. The complete clinical picture and exposure history should be considered, and imaging tests, e.g., chest X-rays, may also be recommended. Workers with fibrotic lung diseases, such as asbestosis, often have an abnormally low FVC and FEV_1, but their FEV_1/FVC will generally be above the LLN.

Mixed Impairment
If both obstruction and possible restriction are present, *mixed impairment* is possible. However, medical personnel should bear in mind that the air-trapping accompanying pronounced airways obstruction often prevents full recording of the FVC. More extensive tests of pulmonary function may be required to determine whether a true mixed impairment pattern exists.

Normal Spirometry Results
If the FEV_1/FVC is ≥ LLN, there is no obstructive impairment (step 2 of Figure 18). If FVC is also ≥ LLN, there is no restrictive impairment (step 3 of Figure 18), and the worker has *normal spirometry* results.

Since the LLN is defined so that 5 percent of healthy individuals will fall below it, spirometry results from a worker without any apparent health problems are occasionally found to be slightly below the LLN. The worker should be retested at a later date to confirm the results and, if still abnormal, the complete clinical presentation should be evaluated. Additional tests of pulmonary function should be done if clinically indicated (4).

3.1.4 UNDERSTANDING PERCENT OF PREDICTED VALUES

In addition to determining whether a worker falls below the normal range and exhibits possible impairment, the PLHCP may also wish to compare a worker's lung function with the average of the normal range, i.e., the "predicted" values, expected for him/her. When a worker's measured result equals his/her predicted value, it indicates that the worker has average lung function (i.e., 100 percent of predicted). Values below predicted but within the normal range often simply indicate below-average lung function and do not necessarily indicate loss of function. Similarly, high FVC or FEV_1 values indicate above-average lung function when measured by a technically valid test. Many "healthy workers" have lung function that is considerably above average when they begin working. For example, young adults who were competitive athletes while their lungs were still growing may have results above 120 percent of predicted value.

However, it is unusual to have results above 130 percent of predicted value, so if this occurs, check that the worker's age, height, and race-adjustment factor (if used) are correctly entered and that a problem with sensor contamination or an incorrect spirometer calibration does not exist.

3.2 EVALUATING RESULTS OVER TIME

3.2.1 WHY LOOK AT CHANGE OVER TIME?

Adults experience a normal, gradual decline in lung function as they age, but some occupational and personal exposures can accelerate this loss of function over time. Periodic spirometry testing can be used to detect such accelerated losses. To evaluate lung function loss over time, periodic (or "serial") spirometry testing measures baseline lung function, and then compares the baseline to follow-up values measured at later time points. This process is known as "longitudinal evaluation."

Longitudinal evaluation of accurate serial test results can help PLHCPs make decisions about worker respiratory health or the need for medical referrals. Longitudinal evaluation may be especially important for workers who have above-average lung function (i.e., >100 percent of predicted). Such workers' lung function may decline over time from the top to the bottom of the normal range, without dropping below their LLN. Although such declines may not be detected by repeatedly determining whether the results from single examinations are within the worker's current normal range, these declines – which may indicate a significant loss of lung function – may be detected by longitudinal evaluation. In addition, careful monitoring of longitudinal results from groups of workers in a workplace may indicate that exposures to known respiratory hazards need to be reduced. Such group evaluations might also help to identify previously unrecognized occupational hazards.

However, these benefits of longitudinal evaluation can only be realized if extraneous measurement variability is kept to a minimum. If the variability associated with spirometry testing is much larger than the actual loss of lung function over time, it will reduce the ability to accurately detect and interpret lung function losses. For example, a falsely elevated baseline value can make declines appear excessive, or a falsely low baseline result can mask a significant loss of function. Therefore, technicians who perform serial spirometry testing and PLHCPs who evaluate those results should be especially aware of and hold constant the technical and biological factors that will affect spirometry test results over time. The pitfalls to be avoided in longitudinal evaluation are discussed below.

3.2.2 TECHNICAL AND BIOLOGICAL FACTORS

Variability in serial spirometry results is caused by technical and biological factors. Technical factors include testing techniques, technician competence, and variations in equipment and operating conditions. Biological factors are related to the worker who is being tested and can include circadian rhythms and conditions such as illness or recovery from surgery.

Technical variability in serial testing can be reduced by standardizing and documenting spirometry test procedures and type of equipment used, maintaining equipment, and performing quality assurance (QA) reviews. Standardization of equipment and procedures is especially important if spirometry testing is performed by multiple testing providers (e.g., medical clinics hired by the employer) over time. Variability introduced by frequently changing spirometry providers or using providers that perform poor quality testing will likely make it impossible to accurately measure a worker's change in pulmonary function over time. Records from spirometer accuracy checks, whether performed "in house" or contracted out, should be saved indefinitely, to allow for future troubleshooting of problematic spirometry test results.

Because consistent policies and procedures are essential for high quality and standardized spirometry testing, OSHA recommends that PLHCPs prepare a written testing protocol (i.e., a Spirometry Procedure Manual) and make sure that technicians understand and follow the protocol. As ACOEM notes "the many details involved in conducting tests and maintaining equipment may be easily misunderstood, resulting in non-standardized testing procedures" (6). Details of what should be included in the manual and how it should be used are presented below in the Spirometry Procedure Manual section.

Critical factors to consider when conducting serial spirometry testing are summarized in Table 1, below.

3.2.3 FREQUENCY OF TESTING

Factors to consider when determining the frequency of serial testing are: (1) the severity of the lung disease that could develop; (2) how well it has been demonstrated that rate of lung function decline predicts disease development; (3) the effectiveness of interventions or treatments on disease outcome; and (4) OSHA requirements that apply when testing workers exposed to regulated substances such as asbestos, coke oven emissions, cotton dust, cadmium, formaldehyde, and benzene (see 29 CFR 1910.1001, 1910.1029, 1910.1043, 1910.1027, 1910.1048, and 1910.1028). These factors and, therefore the frequency of testing, are likely to vary depending on the specific exposures and diseases under consideration. Assistance from a pulmonary or occupational physician specialist, if not the PLHCP, may be needed to determine the likely course of potential lung function decline and the efficacy of medical intervention on impairment and disease outcome.

3.2.4 VALUES THAT SUGGEST ABNORMALITY

Unlike the method for comparing a worker's test results with his/her reference values at one point in time, discussed above, no strong agreement exists on what constitutes an excessive loss of lung

Table 1. Critical Factors When Conducting Spirometry Testing Over Time

1. Standardize and document the testing protocol, equipment used, and all protocol or equipment changes.

2. Provide technicians with initial and periodic training, and periodically audit technical quality of spirograms (QA reviews).

3. Maintain equipment

    - Avoid unneeded equipment changes.

    - Avoid unnecessary changes in spirometer configuration.

    - Verify spirometer accuracy.

        a. Obtain evidence of validation testing of spirometer from the manufacturer

        b. Check calibration at least daily during use

        c. Routinely evaluate technical quality of spirograms and patterns of test results

    - Save calibration records for as long as needed to support accuracy of spirometry results.

4. Minimize biological variability

    - Conduct testing in same posture as previous tests (e.g., standing or sitting).

    - Conduct testing at the same time of day and season to assess long-term change.

    - Postpone testing for one hour after smoking, using a bronchodilator, or eating a heavy meal; three days after recovering from an illness that lasted three weeks or less; three weeks after a severe respiratory illness or ear infection; and six or more weeks after eye, ear, chest, or abdominal surgery, unless a surgeon provides a release statement.

Adapted from ACOEM (6).

function over time. A "significant" lung function decline should detect deteriorating lung function at an early stage but avoid false positive findings in workers whose lung function measurements may be variable but are not declining faster than expected.

The ATS/ERS recommends using FEV_1 as the spirometry measurement to evaluate lung function decline over time (4). This measurement is reduced by both obstructive and restrictive changes in lung function, and it is generally unaffected by testing errors such as early termination, which affect the accuracy of the FVC. Because the FEV_1/FVC is affected by factors that impact both the FEV_1 and the FVC, it also is not the outcome of choice when following change in function over time. When too many indices of lung function are tracked simultaneously, the risk of false-positive interpretations of change increases (4).

Aging significantly affects lung function over time, causing gradual decreases in volume of approximately 0.03 L/year, on the average, in non-smoking adults over age 35. Although aging has little impact on lung function loss over short intervals, NIOSH takes aging into account when evaluating serial tests over periods of more than one year (15). A loss of FEV_1 exceeding 15 percent has been regarded as potentially excessive by ACOEM (5, 6), ATS/ERS (4), NIOSH (15), and the California Department of Public Health (16), and should be evaluated, as described below.

The 15 percent criterion should distinguish significant lung function decline from the usual variability in spirometry performance experienced by many spirometry testing programs. However, recent studies by NIOSH indicate that smaller losses, e.g., declines of 8–10 percent, might be considered significant when longitudinal evaluation is applied to standardized high quality serial spirometry test results from healthy workers (17). ACOEM recently stated that declines of 10–15 percent from baseline, after taking aging into account, may be important when known deleterious exposures are considered (5).

3.2.5 INTERPRETING CHANGE OVER TIME

The importance of conducting valid tests and maintaining high technical quality cannot be overstated when evaluating change over time. Therefore, before interpreting spirometry results, the PLHCP should verify technical quality of the testing and reject inadequate tests. The PLHCP should also verify that the follow-up period was adequate since estimates of loss of function become less variable as the length of follow-up increases, and only large losses of lung function can be reliably detected over short time periods (6).

When evaluating a worker's changes in lung function over time, PLHCPs should bear in mind that rates of pulmonary function change are affected by multiple factors. Some of those factors are work-related, e.g., job exposures, while others are non-occupational, e.g., weight gain, habits such as smoking, or pre-existing lung diseases such as asthma. Therefore, determinations of lung function decline should consider the whole clinical presentation in addition to spirometry results.

If a worker is determined to have "excessive" loss of function, two follow-up steps are recommended: (1) technical error should be ruled out by re-evaluating the test results for validity and repeating the spirometry test if needed; and (2) the worker should be referred for further medical evaluation including an assessment of the complete clinical picture and possibly additional tests of pulmonary function.

4.0 QUALITY ASSURANCE (QA) REVIEWS

High quality spirometry tests are essential for correct interpretation and classification of worker respiratory health. If a PLHCP concludes that spirometry results are not reliable, workers may need to be re-tested and the effectiveness of the entire worker monitoring program may be called into question. Therefore, OSHA recommends that facilities conducting occupational spirometry tests establish on-going programs of regular QA reviews of spirograms and calibration check records.

QA reviews should be conducted by individuals experienced in recognizing and correcting flawed spirometry tests, such as a PLHCP, a qualified medical director, or a third-party vendor. Randomly selected test reports, all invalid tests, and a sampling of tests with unusually low or high results (e.g., FEV_1 or FVC below LLN or >130 percent of predicted) should be examined. Though electronic tracings and records are evaluated most efficiently, hard-copy reports can also be reviewed. Reviews should be performed at least quarterly and more often if the technician is inexperienced or if poor technical quality is observed. Reports on test session quality should be prepared monthly, or at least quarterly, for each technician.

After the QA review, feedback to the technician should focus on evaluating his/her coaching skills and understanding of the elements of a valid spirometry test. The technician should also be allowed to provide feedback to the QA reviewer. Periodic discussions between the technician and QA reviewer should include:

1. Frequency and type of technical errors causing unacceptable curves and the frequency of non-repeatable tests;
2. Coaching actions that the technician can take to improve test quality;
3. Positive feedback for good performance;
4. Comments regarding spirometer configuration settings and formatting of reports of test results; and
5. Feedback from the technician about what can be done to improve spirometry results (e.g., providing workers with educational materials or better storage and maintenance of equipment).

The goal is to assure that at least 80 percent of spirometry tests are technically valid (16). Supervision or retraining of a technician is indicated when the overall spirometry test quality falls below an 80 percent success rate.

5.0 SPIROMETRY PROCEDURE MANUAL

The central document in a good spirometry testing program is a written Spirometry Procedure Manual. Such a manual makes spirometry testing procedures and equipment calibration information readily available and ensures that the same standardized procedures are available to all staff and substitute staff. The manual should also be used to help train new staff. The Spirometry Procedure Manual should include:

1. Equipment calibration check procedures, and how often they are performed;
2. A detailed description of the spirometry testing procedures;
3. Criteria for valid tests;
4. Reference values ("predicted normals") source;
5. Protocols established to prevent and correct sensor contamination and zero-flow errors in flow-type spirometers and actions to be taken when flawed values are observed;
6. Required training for personnel involved in spirometry testing program;
7. Protocol for QA reviews;
8. Pre-test eligibility questions;
9. Sample reports;
10. Manufacturer's spirometer user manual and contact information for manufacturer and local distributor;
11. List of necessary supplies;
12. Instructions for infection control procedures, including cleaning or sterilizing the spirometer; and
13. Date and filename for the current version of the procedure manual.

Appendix B of this document contains a checklist for developing the spirometry procedure manual.

6.0 RECORDKEEPING

Adequate recordkeeping is a critical component of a good spirometry program. To improve the quality of spirometry testing programs, OSHA makes recommendations below on three recordkeeping components: (1) Spirometry test reports, (2) Equipment maintenance records, and (3) Personnel training and evaluation records.

1. **Spirometry Test Reports:** OSHA standards require employers to ensure that medical records for each worker, including the spirometry test results, are maintained for at least 30 years following the end of employment (see 29 CFR 1910.1020).

   Spirometry test reports should include:

   a. Test date and time;
   b. Worker's name, identification number, age, height, gender, and race;
   c. Spirometer used (e.g., type, serial number, etc.);
   d. Ambient air or spirometer temperature and barometric pressure, if appropriate;
   e. Test posture used (sitting or standing);
   f. Source of reference values used (for predicted normal and LLN values);
   g. Test results from at least the three best curves, preferably from all recorded maneuvers, with test sequence indicated;
   h. Technician's name or initials;
   i. Technician comments on worker cooperation/effort or other aspects of the test session;
   j. Flow-volume and volume-time curves for all saved efforts, preferably meeting recommended minimum hard-copy graph sizes (Figure 4b);
   k. A measure of repeatability; and
   l. Date of last calibration check.

2. **Equipment Maintenance Records:** Since equipment maintenance records support the accuracy of the spirometry test results in the medical record, OSHA also recommends saving the equipment records described below. Availability of such records permits later troubleshooting of problematic spirometry test results, which is particularly important when conducting periodic spirometry testing.

   Equipment Maintenance Records for each spirometer should include:

   a. A quality control log which records calibration checks, routine maintenance, upgrades, repairs performed and the results, the date and time of each procedure, and the technician's name. Some computerized spirometry systems store this information in a database. Reports generated during calibration checks should be saved indefinitely; and
   b. The model, serial number, and identification number of the spirometer, and dates and versions of computer software and hardware updates or changes. Store the manufacturer's manuals, warranties, etc. with the quality control log.

3. **Personnel Training and Evaluation Records:** OSHA also recommends that personnel qualifications be documented and available for review.

   Personnel Training and Evaluation Records should include:

   a. Records of technician continuing education and results of evaluation and feedback to technicians; and
   b. Certificates from completed NIOSH-approved spirometry training courses.

7.0 REFERENCES

1. Occupational Safety and Health Administration (OSHA). Occupational Exposure to Cotton Dust. 43 Fed. Reg. 27350. July 26, 1978.

2. Miller MR, Crapo R, Hankinson J, Brusasco V, Burgos F, Casaburi R, Coates A, Enright P, van der Grinten CP, Gustafsson P, Jensen R, Johnson DC, MacIntyre N, McKay R, Navajas D, Pedersen OF, Pellegrino R, Viegi G, Wanger J. American Thoracic Society/European Respiratory Society (ATS/ERS) Task Force: General Considerations for Lung Function Testing. Eur Respir J; 26 (1): 153-161, 2005. http://www.thoracic.org/statements/resources/pfet/PFT1.pdf.

3. Miller MR, Hankinson J, Brusasco V, Burgos F, Casaburi R, Coates A, Crapo R, Enright P, van der Grinten CP, Gustafsson P, Jensen R, Johnson DC, MacIntyre N, McKay R, Navajas D, Pedersen OF, Pellegrino R, Viegi G, Wanger J. American Thoracic Society/European Respiratory Society (ATS/ERS) Task Force: Standardisation of Spirometry. Eur Respir J; 26: 319-338, 2005. http://www.thoracic.org/statements/resources/pfet/PFT2.pdf.

4. Pellegrino R, Viegi G, Brusasco V, Crapo RO, Burgos F, Casaburi R, Coates A, van der Grinten CP, Gustafsson P, Hankinson J, Jensen R, Johnson DC, MacIntyre N, McKay R, Miller MR, Navajas D, Pedersen OF, Wanger J. American Thoracic Society/European Respiratory Society (ATS/ERS) Task Force: Interpretative Strategies for Lung Function Tests. Eur Respir J; 26:948-968, 2005. http://www.thoracic.org/statements/resources/pfet/pft5.pdf.

5. Townsend MC. American College of Occupational and Environmental Medicine (ACOEM) Occupational and Environmental Lung Disorders Committee. Spirometry in the Occupational Health Setting—2011 update. J Occup Environ Med; 53:569-584, 2011. http://www.acoem.org/uploadedFiles/Public_Affairs/Policies_And_Position_Statements/ACOEM%20Spirometry%20Statement.pdf.

6. Townsend, MC. American College of Occupational and Environmental Medicine (ACOEM) Position Statement: Evaluating Pulmonary Function Change Over Time in the Occupational Setting. JOEM; 47:1307-1316, 2005.

7. Townsend, MC. American College of Occupational and Environmental Medicine (ACOEM) Position Statement: Spirometry in the Occupational Setting. JOEM; 42:228-245, 2000.

8. National Institute of Occupational Safety and Health (NIOSH). Spirometry Training Guide. December 1, 2003. http://www.cdc.gov/niosh/docs/2004-154c/pdfs/2004-154c.pdf.

9. International Standards Organization. Anaesthetic and Respiratory Equipment -- Spirometers Intended for the Measurement of Time Forced Expired Volumes in Humans. ISO 26782:2009. Available thorough American National Standards Institute (ANSI) at: http://webstore.ansi.org/RecordDetail.aspx?sku=ISO+26782%3A2009.

10. Townsend MC, Hankinson JL, Lindesmith LA, Slivka WA, Stiver G, Ayres GT. Is My Lung Function Really That Good? Flow-type Spirometer Problems that Elevate Test Results. Chest; 125:1902-1909, 2004. http://www.chestjournal.org/cgi/reprint/125/5/1902.pdf.

11. National Institute for Occupational Safety and Health (NIOSH). U.S. Department of Health and Human Services, Centers for Disease Control and Prevention, Get Valid Spirometry Results Every Time. DHHS (NIOSH) Publication No. 2011-135, 2011.

12. Hankinson JL, Odencrantz JR, Fedan KB. Spirometric Reference Values from a Sample of the General U.S. Population. Am J Resp Crit Care Med; 159:179-187, 1999. http://ajrccm.atsjournals.org/cgi/reprint/159/1/179.pdf.

13. Knudson RJ, Slatin RC, Lebowitz MD, Burrows B. The Maximal Expiratory Flow-Volume Curve. Normal standards, variability, and effects of age. Am Rev Respir Dis; 113:587–600, 1976.

14. Hankinson JL, Kawut SM, Shahar E, Smith LJ, Stukovsky KH, Barr RG. Performance of American Thoracic Society-Recommended Spirometry Reference Values in a Multiethnic Sample of Adults: The Multiethnic Study of Atherosclerosis (MESA) Lung Study. Chest; 137(1):138-45, 2010.

15. National Institute of Occupational Safety and Health (NIOSH). Criteria for a Recommended Standard: Occupational Exposure to Respirable Coal Mine Dust. September 1995.

16. California Department of Public Health. Medical Surveillance for Flavorings-Related Lung Disease Among Flavor Manufacturing Workers in California, August 2007. http://www.cdph.ca.gov/programs/ohb/Documents/flavor-guidelines.pdf.

17. Wang ML, Petsonk E. Repeated Measures of FEV_1 over Six to Twelve Months: What Change is Abnormal? J Occup Environ Med; 46:591-595, 2004.

APPENDIX A

NATIONAL HEALTH AND NUTRITION EXAMINATION SURVEY III (NHANES III) REFERENCE VALUES

(Tables Generated by NIOSH using Hankinson et al., 1999 prediction equations (12))

FEV$_1$/FVC Ratios (%) - Caucasian Males - NHANES III *

Ratio	\multicolumn{27}{c}{Age}
	18	20	22	24	26	28	30	32	34	36	38	40	42	44	46	48	50	52	54	56	58	60	62	64	66	68	70
Predicted	84.3	83.9	83.5	83.1	82.7	82.3	81.9	81.5	81.0	80.6	80.2	79.8	79.4	79.0	78.6	78.1	77.7	77.3	76.9	76.5	76.1	75.7	75.3	74.8	74.4	74.0	73.6
LLN	74.7	74.3	73.8	73.4	73.0	72.6	72.2	71.8	71.4	71.0	70.5	70.1	69.7	69.3	68.9	68.5	68.1	67.6	67.2	66.8	66.4	66.0	65.6	65.2	64.8	64.3	63.9

FEV$_1$/FVC Ratios (%) - African-American Males - NHANES III *

Ratio	\multicolumn{27}{c}{Age}
	18	20	22	24	26	28	30	32	34	36	38	40	42	44	46	48	50	52	54	56	58	60	62	64	66	68	70
Predicted	85.9	85.6	85.2	84.9	84.5	84.1	83.8	83.4	83.0	82.7	82.3	81.9	81.6	81.2	80.8	80.5	80.1	79.7	79.4	79.0	78.6	78.3	77.9	77.5	77.2	76.8	76.4
LLN	75.5	75.2	74.8	74.4	74.1	73.7	73.3	73.0	72.6	72.2	71.9	71.5	71.1	70.8	70.4	70.0	69.7	69.3	69.0	68.6	68.2	67.9	67.5	67.1	66.8	66.4	66.0

FEV$_1$/FVC Ratios (%) - Mexican-American Males - NHANES III *

Ratio	\multicolumn{27}{c}{Age}
	18	20	22	24	26	28	30	32	34	36	38	40	42	44	46	48	50	52	54	56	58	60	62	64	66	68	70
Predicted	86.1	85.7	85.2	84.8	84.3	83.9	83.5	83.0	82.6	82.2	81.7	81.3	80.8	80.4	80.0	79.5	79.1	78.7	78.2	77.8	77.3	76.9	76.5	76.0	75.6	75.2	74.7
LLN	77.0	76.6	76.1	75.7	75.2	74.8	74.4	73.9	73.5	73.1	72.6	72.2	71.7	71.3	70.9	70.4	70.0	69.6	69.1	68.7	68.2	67.8	67.4	66.9	66.5	66.1	65.6

FEV$_1$/FVC Ratios (%) - Caucasian Females - NHANES III *

Ratio	\multicolumn{27}{c}{Age}
Age	18	20	22	24	26	28	30	32	34	36	38	40	42	44	46	48	50	52	54	56	58	60	62	64	66	68	70
Predicted	87.0	86.6	86.1	85.7	85.3	84.9	84.4	84.0	83.6	83.2	82.7	82.3	81.9	81.5	81.0	80.6	80.2	79.8	79.3	78.9	78.5	78.1	77.6	77.2	76.8	76.4	75.9
LLN	77.2	76.8	76.3	75.9	75.5	75.1	74.6	74.2	73.8	73.4	72.9	72.5	72.1	71.7	71.2	70.8	70.4	70.0	69.5	69.1	68.7	68.3	67.8	67.4	67.0	66.6	66.1

FEV$_1$/FVC Ratios (%) - African-American Females - NHANES III *

Age	18	20	22	24	26	28	30	32	34	36	38	40	42	44	46	48	50	52	54	56	58	60	62	64	66	68	70
Predicted	88.0	87.6	87.2	86.8	86.4	85.9	85.5	85.1	84.7	84.3	83.9	83.5	83.1	82.7	82.3	81.9	81.5	81.1	80.6	80.2	79.8	79.4	79.0	78.6	78.2	77.8	77.4
LLN	77.3	76.9	76.5	76.1	75.7	75.3	74.9	74.5	74.0	73.6	73.2	72.8	72.4	72.0	71.6	71.2	70.8	70.4	70.0	69.6	69.2	68.7	68.3	67.9	67.5	67.1	66.7

FEV$_1$/FVC Ratios (%) - Mexican-American Females - NHANES III *

Age	18	20	22	24	26	28	30	32	34	36	38	40	42	44	46	48	50	52	54	56	58	60	62	64	66	68	70
Predicted	88.3	87.9	87.4	87.0	86.5	86.1	85.6	85.2	84.7	84.3	83.8	83.4	82.9	82.5	82.0	81.6	81.1	80.7	80.2	79.8	79.3	78.9	78.4	78.0	77.5	77.1	76.6
LLN	79.0	78.5	78.1	77.6	77.2	76.7	76.3	75.9	75.4	75.0	74.5	74.1	73.6	73.2	72.7	72.3	71.8	71.4	70.9	70.5	70.0	69.6	69.1	68.7	68.2	67.8	67.3

*The tables are shown by age only, since height does not affect the normal range for FEV$_1$/FVC ratio.

Predicted FVC (L) - Caucasian Males - NHANES III

Height (Inches)	18	20	22	24	26	28	30	32	34	36	38	40	42	44	46	48	50	52	54	56	58	60	62	64	66	68	70
58.0	3.40	3.76	3.74	3.71	3.69	3.66	3.63	3.60	3.56	3.53	3.49	3.45	3.40	3.36	3.31	3.26	3.21	3.16	3.10	3.04	2.98	2.92	2.86	2.79	2.72	2.65	2.58
59.0	3.54	3.90	3.88	3.85	3.83	3.80	3.77	3.74	3.70	3.67	3.63	3.59	3.55	3.50	3.45	3.40	3.35	3.30	3.24	3.19	3.13	3.06	3.00	2.93	2.86	2.79	2.72
60.0	3.68	4.04	4.02	4.00	3.97	3.94	3.91	3.88	3.85	3.81	3.77	3.73	3.69	3.64	3.60	3.55	3.50	3.44	3.39	3.33	3.27	3.21	3.14	3.08	3.01	2.94	2.86
61.0	3.83	4.19	4.17	4.14	4.12	4.09	4.06	4.03	3.99	3.96	3.92	3.88	3.83	3.79	3.74	3.69	3.64	3.59	3.53	3.47	3.41	3.35	3.29	3.22	3.15	3.08	3.01
62.0	3.97	4.34	4.31	4.29	4.26	4.24	4.21	4.17	4.14	4.10	4.07	4.03	3.98	3.94	3.89	3.84	3.79	3.74	3.68	3.62	3.56	3.50	3.44	3.37	3.30	3.23	3.16
63.0	4.12	4.49	4.46	4.44	4.42	4.39	4.36	4.33	4.29	4.25	4.22	4.18	4.13	4.09	4.04	3.99	3.94	3.89	3.83	3.77	3.71	3.65	3.59	3.52	3.45	3.38	3.31
64.0	4.28	4.64	4.62	4.59	4.57	4.54	4.51	4.48	4.44	4.41	4.37	4.33	4.29	4.24	4.19	4.14	4.09	4.04	3.98	3.93	3.87	3.80	3.74	3.67	3.60	3.53	3.46
65.0	4.43	4.79	4.77	4.75	4.72	4.70	4.67	4.63	4.60	4.56	4.52	4.48	4.44	4.40	4.35	4.30	4.25	4.19	4.14	4.08	4.02	3.96	3.89	3.83	3.76	3.69	3.61
66.0	4.59	4.95	4.93	4.91	4.88	4.85	4.82	4.79	4.76	4.72	4.68	4.64	4.60	4.55	4.51	4.46	4.41	4.35	4.30	4.24	4.18	4.12	4.05	3.98	3.92	3.85	3.77
67.0	4.75	5.11	5.09	5.07	5.04	5.01	4.98	4.95	4.92	4.88	4.84	4.80	4.76	4.71	4.67	4.62	4.57	4.51	4.46	4.40	4.34	4.28	4.21	4.14	4.08	4.01	3.93
68.0	4.91	5.27	5.25	5.23	5.20	5.18	5.15	5.11	5.08	5.04	5.00	4.96	4.92	4.88	4.83	4.78	4.73	4.67	4.62	4.56	4.50	4.44	4.37	4.31	4.24	4.17	4.09
69.0	5.08	5.44	5.42	5.39	5.37	5.34	5.31	5.28	5.24	5.21	5.17	5.13	5.09	5.04	4.99	4.94	4.89	4.84	4.78	4.73	4.66	4.60	4.54	4.47	4.40	4.33	4.26
70.0	5.24	5.61	5.58	5.56	5.53	5.51	5.48	5.44	5.41	5.37	5.34	5.30	5.25	5.21	5.16	5.11	5.06	5.01	4.95	4.89	4.83	4.77	4.71	4.64	4.57	4.50	4.43
71.0	5.41	5.77	5.75	5.73	5.70	5.68	5.65	5.61	5.58	5.54	5.51	5.46	5.42	5.38	5.33	5.28	5.23	5.18	5.12	5.06	5.00	4.94	4.88	4.81	4.74	4.67	4.60
72.0	5.58	5.95	5.93	5.90	5.88	5.85	5.82	5.79	5.75	5.72	5.68	5.64	5.59	5.55	5.50	5.45	5.40	5.35	5.29	5.23	5.17	5.11	5.05	4.98	4.91	4.84	4.77
73.0	5.76	6.12	6.10	6.08	6.05	6.02	5.99	5.96	5.93	5.89	5.85	5.81	5.77	5.72	5.68	5.63	5.58	5.52	5.47	5.41	5.35	5.29	5.22	5.16	5.09	5.02	4.94
74.0	5.94	6.30	6.28	6.25	6.23	6.20	6.17	6.14	6.10	6.07	6.03	5.99	5.95	5.90	5.85	5.80	5.75	5.70	5.64	5.58	5.52	5.46	5.40	5.33	5.26	5.19	5.12
75.0	6.12	6.48	6.46	6.43	6.41	6.38	6.35	6.32	6.28	6.25	6.21	6.17	6.12	6.08	6.03	5.98	5.93	5.88	5.82	5.76	5.70	5.64	5.58	5.51	5.44	5.37	5.30
76.0	6.30	6.66	6.64	6.61	6.59	6.56	6.53	6.50	6.46	6.43	6.39	6.35	6.31	6.26	6.21	6.16	6.11	6.06	6.00	5.95	5.89	5.82	5.76	5.69	5.62	5.55	5.48
77.0	6.48	6.84	6.82	6.80	6.77	6.74	6.71	6.68	6.65	6.61	6.57	6.53	6.49	6.44	6.40	6.35	6.30	6.24	6.19	6.13	6.07	6.01	5.94	5.88	5.81	5.74	5.66
78.0	6.67	7.03	7.01	6.98	6.96	6.93	6.90	6.87	6.83	6.80	6.76	6.72	6.68	6.63	6.58	6.53	6.48	6.43	6.37	6.32	6.26	6.19	6.13	6.06	5.99	5.92	5.85
79.0	6.86	7.22	7.20	7.17	7.15	7.12	7.09	7.06	7.02	6.99	6.95	6.91	6.87	6.82	6.77	6.72	6.67	6.62	6.56	6.51	6.45	6.38	6.32	6.25	6.18	6.11	6.04
80.0	7.05	7.41	7.39	7.36	7.34	7.31	7.28	7.25	7.21	7.18	7.14	7.10	7.06	7.01	6.96	6.91	6.86	6.81	6.75	6.70	6.64	6.57	6.51	6.44	6.37	6.30	6.23

LLN for FVC (L) - Caucasian Males - NHANES III

Height (Inches)	18	20	22	24	26	28	30	32	34	36	38	40	42	44	46	48	50	52	54	56	58	60	62	64	66	68	70
58.0	2.76	3.12	3.10	3.07	3.05	3.02	2.99	2.96	2.92	2.89	2.85	2.81	2.77	2.72	2.67	2.62	2.57	2.52	2.46	2.41	2.35	2.28	2.22	2.15	2.08	2.01	1.94
59.0	2.87	3.24	3.22	3.19	3.17	3.14	3.11	3.08	3.04	3.01	2.97	2.93	2.88	2.84	2.79	2.74	2.69	2.64	2.58	2.52	2.46	2.40	2.34	2.27	2.20	2.13	2.06
60.0	3.00	3.36	3.34	3.31	3.29	3.26	3.23	3.20	3.16	3.13	3.09	3.05	3.00	2.96	2.91	2.86	2.81	2.76	2.70	2.64	2.58	2.52	2.46	2.39	2.32	2.25	2.18
61.0	3.12	3.48	3.46	3.43	3.41	3.38	3.35	3.32	3.29	3.25	3.21	3.17	3.13	3.08	3.03	2.99	2.93	2.88	2.82	2.77	2.71	2.64	2.58	2.51	2.44	2.37	2.30
62.0	3.24	3.60	3.58	3.56	3.53	3.51	3.48	3.44	3.41	3.37	3.33	3.29	3.25	3.21	3.16	3.11	3.06	3.00	2.95	2.89	2.83	2.77	2.70	2.64	2.57	2.50	2.43
63.0	3.37	3.73	3.71	3.69	3.66	3.63	3.60	3.57	3.54	3.50	3.46	3.42	3.38	3.33	3.29	3.24	3.19	3.13	3.08	3.02	2.96	2.90	2.83	2.76	2.70	2.63	2.55
64.0	3.50	3.86	3.84	3.81	3.79	3.76	3.73	3.70	3.67	3.63	3.59	3.55	3.51	3.46	3.41	3.37	3.31	3.26	3.20	3.15	3.09	3.02	2.96	2.89	2.82	2.75	2.68
65.0	3.63	3.99	3.97	3.95	3.92	3.89	3.86	3.83	3.80	3.76	3.72	3.68	3.64	3.59	3.55	3.50	3.44	3.39	3.34	3.28	3.22	3.15	3.09	3.02	2.96	2.88	2.81
66.0	3.76	4.12	4.10	4.08	4.05	4.02	3.99	3.96	3.93	3.89	3.85	3.81	3.77	3.72	3.68	3.63	3.58	3.52	3.47	3.41	3.35	3.29	3.22	3.16	3.09	3.02	2.94
67.0	3.90	4.26	4.24	4.21	4.19	4.16	4.13	4.10	4.06	4.03	3.99	3.95	3.90	3.86	3.81	3.76	3.71	3.66	3.60	3.54	3.48	3.42	3.36	3.29	3.22	3.15	3.08
68.0	4.03	4.39	4.37	4.35	4.32	4.30	4.27	4.23	4.20	4.16	4.12	4.08	4.04	4.00	3.95	3.90	3.85	3.79	3.74	3.68	3.62	3.56	3.49	3.43	3.36	3.29	3.22
69.0	4.17	4.53	4.51	4.49	4.46	4.43	4.40	4.37	4.34	4.30	4.26	4.22	4.18	4.13	4.09	4.04	3.99	3.93	3.88	3.82	3.76	3.70	3.63	3.57	3.50	3.43	3.35
70.0	4.31	4.67	4.65	4.63	4.60	4.58	4.55	4.51	4.48	4.44	4.40	4.36	4.32	4.28	4.23	4.18	4.13	4.07	4.02	3.96	3.90	3.84	3.77	3.71	3.64	3.57	3.50
71.0	4.45	4.82	4.79	4.77	4.75	4.72	4.69	4.66	4.62	4.59	4.55	4.51	4.46	4.42	4.37	4.32	4.27	4.22	4.16	4.10	4.04	3.98	3.92	3.85	3.78	3.71	3.64
72.0	4.60	4.96	4.94	4.92	4.89	4.86	4.83	4.80	4.77	4.73	4.69	4.65	4.61	4.56	4.52	4.47	4.42	4.36	4.31	4.25	4.19	4.13	4.06	4.00	3.93	3.86	3.78
73.0	4.75	5.11	5.09	5.06	5.04	5.01	4.98	4.95	4.91	4.88	4.84	4.80	4.76	4.71	4.66	4.61	4.56	4.51	4.45	4.39	4.33	4.27	4.21	4.14	4.07	4.00	3.93
74.0	4.89	5.26	5.24	5.21	5.19	5.16	5.13	5.10	5.06	5.03	4.99	4.95	4.90	4.86	4.81	4.76	4.71	4.66	4.60	4.54	4.48	4.42	4.36	4.29	4.22	4.15	4.08
75.0	5.05	5.41	5.39	5.36	5.34	5.31	5.28	5.25	5.21	5.18	5.14	5.10	5.05	5.01	4.96	4.91	4.86	4.81	4.75	4.69	4.63	4.57	4.51	4.44	4.37	4.30	4.23
76.0	5.20	5.56	5.54	5.52	5.49	5.46	5.43	5.40	5.37	5.33	5.29	5.25	5.21	5.16	5.12	5.07	5.01	4.96	4.91	4.85	4.79	4.73	4.66	4.59	4.53	4.46	4.38
77.0	5.35	5.72	5.69	5.67	5.65	5.62	5.59	5.56	5.52	5.48	5.45	5.41	5.36	5.32	5.27	5.22	5.17	5.12	5.06	5.00	4.94	4.88	4.82	4.75	4.68	4.61	4.54
78.0	5.51	5.87	5.85	5.83	5.80	5.77	5.74	5.71	5.68	5.64	5.60	5.56	5.52	5.47	5.43	5.38	5.33	5.27	5.22	5.16	5.10	5.04	4.97	4.91	4.84	4.77	4.69
79.0	5.67	6.03	6.01	5.99	5.96	5.93	5.90	5.87	5.84	5.80	5.76	5.72	5.68	5.63	5.59	5.54	5.49	5.43	5.38	5.32	5.26	5.20	5.13	5.07	5.00	4.93	4.85
80.0	5.83	6.19	6.17	6.15	6.12	6.09	6.06	6.03	6.00	5.96	5.92	5.88	5.84	5.79	5.75	5.70	5.65	5.59	5.54	5.48	5.42	5.36	5.29	5.23	5.16	5.09	5.01

Predicted FEV₁ (L) - Caucasian Males - NHANES III

Height (Inches)	18	20	22	24	26	28	30	32	34	36	38	40	42	44	46	48	50	52	54	56	58	60	62	64	66	68	70
58.0	3.03	3.28	3.24	3.20	3.16	3.11	3.07	3.02	2.97	2.92	2.87	2.82	2.76	2.71	2.65	2.59	2.53	2.47	2.41	2.34	2.28	2.21	2.14	2.07	2.00	1.93	1.86
59.0	3.13	3.39	3.35	3.31	3.26	3.22	3.17	3.13	3.08	3.03	2.98	2.92	2.87	2.81	2.76	2.70	2.64	2.58	2.51	2.45	2.39	2.32	2.25	2.18	2.11	2.04	1.96
60.0	3.24	3.50	3.46	3.42	3.37	3.33	3.28	3.23	3.19	3.14	3.08	3.03	2.98	2.92	2.86	2.81	2.75	2.69	2.62	2.56	2.49	2.43	2.36	2.29	2.22	2.15	2.07
61.0	3.35	3.61	3.57	3.53	3.48	3.44	3.39	3.34	3.30	3.25	3.19	3.14	3.09	3.03	2.97	2.92	2.86	2.80	2.73	2.67	2.60	2.54	2.47	2.40	2.33	2.26	2.18
62.0	3.46	3.72	3.68	3.64	3.59	3.55	3.50	3.46	3.41	3.36	3.31	3.25	3.20	3.14	3.09	3.03	2.97	2.91	2.84	2.78	2.72	2.65	2.58	2.51	2.44	2.37	2.29
63.0	3.58	3.83	3.79	3.75	3.71	3.66	3.62	3.57	3.52	3.47	3.42	3.37	3.31	3.26	3.20	3.14	3.08	3.02	2.96	2.89	2.83	2.76	2.69	2.63	2.55	2.48	2.41
64.0	3.69	3.95	3.91	3.87	3.82	3.78	3.73	3.69	3.64	3.59	3.54	3.48	3.43	3.37	3.32	3.26	3.20	3.14	3.07	3.01	2.94	2.88	2.81	2.74	2.67	2.60	2.52
65.0	3.81	4.07	4.03	3.98	3.94	3.90	3.85	3.80	3.75	3.70	3.65	3.60	3.55	3.49	3.43	3.37	3.31	3.25	3.19	3.13	3.06	3.00	2.93	2.86	2.79	2.72	2.64
66.0	3.93	4.19	4.15	4.10	4.06	4.02	3.97	3.92	3.87	3.82	3.77	3.72	3.66	3.61	3.55	3.49	3.43	3.37	3.31	3.25	3.18	3.11	3.05	2.98	2.91	2.83	2.76
67.0	4.05	4.31	4.27	4.22	4.18	4.14	4.09	4.04	3.99	3.94	3.89	3.84	3.79	3.73	3.67	3.61	3.56	3.49	3.43	3.37	3.30	3.24	3.17	3.10	3.03	2.96	2.88
68.0	4.17	4.43	4.39	4.35	4.30	4.26	4.21	4.17	4.12	4.07	4.02	3.96	3.91	3.85	3.80	3.74	3.68	3.62	3.55	3.49	3.42	3.36	3.29	3.22	3.15	3.08	3.00
69.0	4.30	4.55	4.51	4.47	4.43	4.38	4.34	4.29	4.24	4.19	4.14	4.09	4.03	3.98	3.92	3.86	3.80	3.74	3.68	3.61	3.55	3.48	3.41	3.35	3.27	3.20	3.13
70.0	4.42	4.68	4.64	4.60	4.56	4.51	4.46	4.42	4.37	4.32	4.27	4.21	4.16	4.10	4.05	3.99	3.93	3.87	3.81	3.74	3.68	3.61	3.54	3.47	3.40	3.33	3.26
71.0	4.55	4.81	4.77	4.73	4.68	4.64	4.59	4.55	4.50	4.45	4.40	4.34	4.29	4.23	4.18	4.12	4.06	4.00	3.93	3.87	3.80	3.74	3.67	3.60	3.53	3.46	3.38
72.0	4.68	4.94	4.90	4.86	4.81	4.77	4.72	4.68	4.63	4.58	4.53	4.47	4.42	4.36	4.31	4.25	4.19	4.13	4.06	4.00	3.93	3.87	3.80	3.73	3.66	3.59	3.51
73.0	4.81	5.07	5.03	4.99	4.95	4.90	4.85	4.81	4.76	4.71	4.66	4.60	4.55	4.49	4.44	4.38	4.32	4.26	4.20	4.13	4.07	4.00	3.93	3.86	3.79	3.72	3.65
74.0	4.95	5.20	5.16	5.12	5.08	5.03	4.99	4.94	4.89	4.84	4.79	4.74	4.68	4.63	4.57	4.51	4.45	4.39	4.33	4.27	4.20	4.13	4.07	4.00	3.93	3.85	3.78
75.0	5.08	5.34	5.30	5.26	5.21	5.17	5.12	5.08	5.03	4.98	4.93	4.87	4.82	4.76	4.71	4.65	4.59	4.53	4.46	4.40	4.34	4.27	4.20	4.13	4.06	3.99	3.91
76.0	5.22	5.48	5.44	5.40	5.35	5.31	5.26	5.21	5.17	5.12	5.06	5.01	4.96	4.90	4.84	4.79	4.73	4.66	4.60	4.54	4.47	4.41	4.34	4.27	4.20	4.13	4.05
77.0	5.36	5.62	5.58	5.53	5.49	5.45	5.40	5.35	5.30	5.25	5.20	5.15	5.10	5.04	4.98	4.92	4.86	4.80	4.74	4.68	4.61	4.55	4.48	4.41	4.34	4.26	4.19
78.0	5.50	5.76	5.72	5.68	5.63	5.59	5.54	5.49	5.45	5.40	5.34	5.29	5.24	5.18	5.12	5.07	5.01	4.94	4.88	4.82	4.75	4.69	4.62	4.55	4.48	4.41	4.33
79.0	5.64	5.90	5.86	5.82	5.78	5.73	5.68	5.64	5.59	5.54	5.49	5.43	5.38	5.32	5.27	5.21	5.15	5.09	5.02	4.96	4.90	4.83	4.76	4.69	4.62	4.55	4.48
80.0	5.79	6.05	6.00	5.96	5.92	5.88	5.83	5.78	5.73	5.68	5.63	5.58	5.52	5.47	5.41	5.35	5.29	5.23	5.17	5.11	5.04	4.97	4.91	4.84	4.77	4.69	4.62

LLN for FEV₁ (L) - Caucasian Males - NHANES III

Height (Inches)	18	20	22	24	26	28	30	32	34	36	38	40	42	44	46	48	50	52	54	56	58	60	62	64	66	68	70
58.0	2.49	2.74	2.70	2.66	2.62	2.57	2.53	2.48	2.43	2.38	2.33	2.28	2.22	2.17	2.11	2.05	1.99	1.93	1.87	1.80	1.74	1.67	1.60	1.53	1.46	1.39	1.32
59.0	2.57	2.83	2.79	2.75	2.71	2.66	2.61	2.57	2.52	2.47	2.42	2.36	2.31	2.25	2.20	2.14	2.08	2.02	1.96	1.89	1.83	1.76	1.69	1.62	1.55	1.48	1.41
60.0	2.66	2.92	2.88	2.84	2.79	2.75	2.70	2.66	2.61	2.56	2.51	2.45	2.40	2.34	2.29	2.23	2.17	2.11	2.04	1.98	1.92	1.85	1.78	1.71	1.64	1.57	1.49
61.0	2.75	3.01	2.97	2.93	2.88	2.84	2.79	2.75	2.70	2.65	2.60	2.54	2.49	2.43	2.38	2.32	2.26	2.20	2.13	2.07	2.01	1.94	1.87	1.80	1.73	1.66	1.59
62.0	2.84	3.10	3.06	3.02	2.98	2.93	2.89	2.84	2.79	2.74	2.69	2.64	2.58	2.53	2.47	2.41	2.35	2.29	2.23	2.16	2.10	2.03	1.96	1.89	1.82	1.75	1.68
63.0	2.94	3.20	3.16	3.11	3.07	3.03	2.98	2.93	2.88	2.83	2.78	2.73	2.68	2.62	2.56	2.50	2.44	2.38	2.32	2.26	2.19	2.12	2.06	1.99	1.92	1.84	1.77
64.0	3.03	3.29	3.25	3.21	3.17	3.12	3.08	3.03	2.98	2.93	2.88	2.82	2.77	2.71	2.66	2.60	2.54	2.48	2.42	2.35	2.29	2.22	2.15	2.08	2.01	1.94	1.87
65.0	3.13	3.39	3.35	3.31	3.26	3.22	3.17	3.12	3.08	3.03	2.97	2.92	2.87	2.81	2.75	2.70	2.64	2.57	2.51	2.45	2.38	2.32	2.25	2.18	2.11	2.04	1.96
66.0	3.23	3.49	3.45	3.40	3.36	3.32	3.27	3.22	3.17	3.12	3.07	3.02	2.96	2.91	2.85	2.79	2.73	2.67	2.61	2.55	2.48	2.41	2.35	2.28	2.21	2.13	2.06
67.0	3.33	3.59	3.55	3.50	3.46	3.42	3.37	3.32	3.27	3.22	3.17	3.12	3.06	3.01	2.95	2.89	2.83	2.77	2.71	2.65	2.58	2.51	2.45	2.38	2.31	2.23	2.16
68.0	3.43	3.69	3.65	3.60	3.56	3.52	3.47	3.42	3.37	3.32	3.27	3.22	3.17	3.11	3.05	2.99	2.93	2.87	2.81	2.75	2.68	2.62	2.55	2.48	2.41	2.33	2.26
69.0	3.53	3.79	3.75	3.71	3.66	3.62	3.57	3.53	3.48	3.43	3.38	3.32	3.27	3.21	3.16	3.10	3.04	2.98	2.91	2.85	2.78	2.72	2.65	2.58	2.51	2.44	2.36
70.0	3.64	3.89	3.85	3.81	3.77	3.72	3.68	3.63	3.58	3.53	3.48	3.43	3.37	3.32	3.26	3.20	3.14	3.08	3.02	2.95	2.89	2.82	2.75	2.68	2.61	2.54	2.47
71.0	3.74	4.00	3.96	3.92	3.87	3.83	3.78	3.74	3.69	3.64	3.58	3.53	3.48	3.42	3.37	3.31	3.25	3.19	3.12	3.06	2.99	2.93	2.86	2.79	2.72	2.65	2.57
72.0	3.85	4.11	4.07	4.02	3.98	3.94	3.89	3.84	3.79	3.74	3.69	3.64	3.58	3.53	3.47	3.41	3.35	3.29	3.23	3.17	3.10	3.03	2.97	2.90	2.83	2.75	2.68
73.0	3.96	4.21	4.17	4.13	4.09	4.04	4.00	3.95	3.90	3.85	3.80	3.75	3.69	3.64	3.58	3.52	3.46	3.40	3.34	3.28	3.21	3.14	3.08	3.01	2.93	2.86	2.79
74.0	4.07	4.32	4.28	4.24	4.20	4.15	4.11	4.06	4.01	3.96	3.91	3.86	3.80	3.75	3.69	3.63	3.57	3.51	3.45	3.39	3.32	3.25	3.19	3.12	3.05	2.97	2.90
75.0	4.18	4.44	4.40	4.35	4.31	4.27	4.22	4.17	4.12	4.07	4.02	3.97	3.92	3.86	3.80	3.74	3.68	3.62	3.56	3.50	3.43	3.36	3.30	3.23	3.16	3.08	3.01
76.0	4.29	4.55	4.51	4.47	4.42	4.38	4.33	4.29	4.24	4.19	4.14	4.08	4.03	3.97	3.92	3.86	3.80	3.74	3.67	3.61	3.54	3.48	3.41	3.34	3.27	3.20	3.12
77.0	4.41	4.66	4.62	4.58	4.54	4.49	4.45	4.40	4.35	4.30	4.25	4.20	4.14	4.09	4.03	3.97	3.91	3.85	3.79	3.72	3.66	3.59	3.52	3.46	3.38	3.31	3.24
78.0	4.52	4.78	4.74	4.70	4.65	4.61	4.56	4.52	4.47	4.42	4.37	4.31	4.26	4.20	4.15	4.09	4.03	3.97	3.90	3.84	3.78	3.71	3.64	3.57	3.50	3.43	3.35
79.0	4.64	4.90	4.86	4.82	4.77	4.73	4.68	4.63	4.59	4.54	4.48	4.43	4.38	4.32	4.26	4.21	4.15	4.08	4.02	3.96	3.89	3.83	3.76	3.69	3.62	3.55	3.47
80.0	4.76	5.02	4.98	4.93	4.89	4.85	4.80	4.75	4.70	4.65	4.60	4.55	4.50	4.44	4.38	4.32	4.26	4.20	4.14	4.08	4.01	3.95	3.88	3.81	3.74	3.66	3.59

Predicted FVC (L) - African American Males - NHANES III

Height (Inches)	Age																											
	18	20	22	24	26	28	30	32	34	36	38	40	42	44	46	48	50	52	54	56	58	60	62	64	66	68	70
60.0	3.07	3.35	3.31	3.28	3.24	3.20	3.17	3.13	3.09	3.06	3.02	2.99	2.95	2.91	2.88	2.84	2.80	2.77	2.73	2.69	2.66	2.62	2.58	2.55	2.51	2.48	2.44
61.0	3.20	3.48	3.44	3.41	3.37	3.33	3.30	3.26	3.22	3.19	3.15	3.12	3.08	3.04	3.01	2.97	2.93	2.90	2.86	2.82	2.79	2.75	2.71	2.68	2.64	2.61	2.57
62.0	3.34	3.61	3.58	3.54	3.50	3.47	3.43	3.39	3.36	3.32	3.28	3.25	3.21	3.17	3.14	3.10	3.07	3.03	2.99	2.96	2.92	2.88	2.85	2.81	2.77	2.74	2.70
63.0	3.47	3.75	3.71	3.67	3.64	3.60	3.56	3.53	3.49	3.45	3.42	3.38	3.35	3.31	3.27	3.24	3.20	3.16	3.13	3.09	3.05	3.02	2.98	2.94	2.91	2.87	2.84
64.0	3.61	3.88	3.85	3.81	3.77	3.74	3.70	3.66	3.63	3.59	3.55	3.52	3.48	3.45	3.41	3.37	3.34	3.30	3.26	3.23	3.19	3.15	3.12	3.08	3.04	3.01	2.97
65.0	3.75	4.02	3.98	3.95	3.91	3.87	3.84	3.80	3.77	3.73	3.69	3.66	3.62	3.58	3.55	3.51	3.47	3.44	3.40	3.37	3.33	3.29	3.26	3.22	3.18	3.15	3.11
66.0	3.89	4.16	4.12	4.09	4.05	4.02	3.98	3.94	3.91	3.87	3.83	3.80	3.76	3.72	3.69	3.65	3.62	3.58	3.54	3.51	3.47	3.43	3.40	3.36	3.32	3.29	3.25
67.0	4.03	4.30	4.27	4.23	4.19	4.16	4.12	4.09	4.05	4.01	3.98	3.94	3.90	3.87	3.83	3.79	3.76	3.72	3.68	3.65	3.61	3.58	3.54	3.50	3.47	3.43	3.39
68.0	4.17	4.45	4.41	4.38	4.34	4.30	4.27	4.23	4.19	4.16	4.12	4.08	4.05	4.01	3.98	3.94	3.90	3.87	3.83	3.79	3.76	3.72	3.68	3.65	3.61	3.57	3.54
69.0	4.32	4.60	4.56	4.52	4.49	4.45	4.41	4.38	4.34	4.30	4.27	4.23	4.20	4.16	4.12	4.09	4.05	4.01	3.98	3.94	3.90	3.87	3.83	3.79	3.76	3.72	3.69
70.0	4.47	4.75	4.71	4.67	4.64	4.60	4.56	4.53	4.49	4.45	4.42	4.38	4.34	4.31	4.27	4.24	4.20	4.16	4.13	4.09	4.05	4.02	3.98	3.94	3.91	3.87	3.83
71.0	4.62	4.90	4.86	4.82	4.79	4.75	4.71	4.68	4.64	4.61	4.57	4.53	4.50	4.46	4.42	4.39	4.35	4.31	4.28	4.24	4.20	4.17	4.13	4.10	4.06	4.02	3.99
72.0	4.77	5.05	5.01	4.98	4.94	4.90	4.87	4.83	4.80	4.76	4.72	4.69	4.65	4.61	4.58	4.54	4.50	4.47	4.43	4.39	4.36	4.32	4.29	4.25	4.21	4.18	4.14
73.0	4.93	5.21	5.17	5.13	5.10	5.06	5.02	4.99	4.95	4.91	4.88	4.84	4.81	4.77	4.73	4.70	4.66	4.62	4.59	4.55	4.51	4.48	4.44	4.40	4.37	4.33	4.30
74.0	5.09	5.36	5.33	5.29	5.25	5.22	5.18	5.15	5.11	5.07	5.04	5.00	4.96	4.93	4.89	4.85	4.82	4.78	4.74	4.71	4.67	4.64	4.60	4.56	4.53	4.49	4.45
75.0	5.25	5.52	5.49	5.45	5.41	5.38	5.34	5.31	5.27	5.23	5.20	5.16	5.12	5.09	5.05	5.01	4.98	4.94	4.90	4.87	4.83	4.80	4.76	4.72	4.69	4.65	4.61
76.0	5.41	5.69	5.65	5.61	5.58	5.54	5.50	5.47	5.43	5.39	5.36	5.32	5.29	5.25	5.21	5.18	5.14	5.10	5.07	5.03	4.99	4.96	4.92	4.88	4.85	4.81	4.78
77.0	5.57	5.85	5.81	5.78	5.74	5.70	5.67	5.63	5.60	5.56	5.52	5.49	5.45	5.41	5.38	5.34	5.30	5.27	5.23	5.19	5.16	5.12	5.09	5.05	5.01	4.98	4.94
78.0	5.74	6.02	5.98	5.94	5.91	5.87	5.83	5.80	5.76	5.73	5.69	5.65	5.62	5.58	5.54	5.51	5.47	5.43	5.40	5.36	5.32	5.29	5.25	5.22	5.18	5.14	5.11
79.0	5.91	6.19	6.15	6.11	6.08	6.04	6.00	5.97	5.93	5.89	5.86	5.82	5.78	5.75	5.71	5.68	5.64	5.60	5.57	5.53	5.49	5.46	5.42	5.38	5.35	5.31	5.27

LLN for FVC (L) - African American Males - NHANES III

Height (Inches)	Age																											
	18	20	22	24	26	28	30	32	34	36	38	40	42	44	46	48	50	52	54	56	58	60	62	64	66	68	70
60.0	2.38	2.66	2.62	2.59	2.55	2.51	2.48	2.44	2.40	2.37	2.33	2.29	2.26	2.22	2.19	2.15	2.11	2.08	2.04	2.00	1.97	1.93	1.89	1.86	1.82	1.78	1.75
61.0	2.49	2.77	2.73	2.69	2.66	2.62	2.58	2.55	2.51	2.47	2.44	2.40	2.37	2.33	2.29	2.26	2.22	2.18	2.15	2.11	2.07	2.04	2.00	1.96	1.93	1.89	1.86
62.0	2.60	2.87	2.84	2.80	2.76	2.73	2.69	2.66	2.62	2.58	2.55	2.51	2.47	2.44	2.40	2.36	2.33	2.29	2.26	2.22	2.18	2.15	2.11	2.07	2.04	2.00	1.96
63.0	2.71	2.98	2.95	2.91	2.88	2.84	2.80	2.77	2.73	2.69	2.66	2.62	2.58	2.55	2.51	2.47	2.44	2.40	2.37	2.33	2.29	2.26	2.22	2.18	2.15	2.11	2.07
64.0	2.82	3.10	3.06	3.02	2.99	2.95	2.91	2.88	2.84	2.81	2.77	2.73	2.70	2.66	2.62	2.59	2.55	2.51	2.48	2.44	2.40	2.37	2.33	2.30	2.26	2.22	2.19
65.0	2.93	3.21	3.17	3.14	3.10	3.06	3.03	2.99	2.96	2.92	2.88	2.85	2.81	2.77	2.74	2.70	2.66	2.63	2.59	2.55	2.52	2.48	2.45	2.41	2.37	2.34	2.30
66.0	3.05	3.33	3.29	3.25	3.22	3.18	3.14	3.11	3.07	3.03	3.00	2.96	2.93	2.89	2.85	2.82	2.78	2.74	2.71	2.67	2.63	2.60	2.56	2.52	2.49	2.45	2.42
67.0	3.17	3.44	3.41	3.37	3.33	3.30	3.26	3.22	3.19	3.15	3.12	3.08	3.04	3.01	2.97	2.93	2.90	2.86	2.82	2.79	2.75	2.71	2.68	2.64	2.61	2.57	2.53
68.0	3.29	3.56	3.53	3.49	3.45	3.42	3.38	3.34	3.31	3.27	3.23	3.20	3.16	3.13	3.09	3.05	3.02	2.98	2.94	2.91	2.87	2.83	2.80	2.76	2.72	2.69	2.65
69.0	3.41	3.68	3.65	3.61	3.57	3.54	3.50	3.46	3.43	3.39	3.36	3.32	3.28	3.25	3.21	3.17	3.14	3.10	3.06	3.03	2.99	2.95	2.92	2.88	2.85	2.81	2.77
70.0	3.53	3.81	3.77	3.73	3.70	3.66	3.62	3.59	3.55	3.51	3.48	3.44	3.40	3.37	3.33	3.30	3.26	3.22	3.19	3.15	3.11	3.08	3.04	3.00	2.97	2.93	2.90
71.0	3.65	3.93	3.89	3.86	3.82	3.78	3.75	3.71	3.67	3.64	3.60	3.57	3.53	3.49	3.46	3.42	3.38	3.35	3.31	3.27	3.24	3.20	3.17	3.13	3.09	3.06	3.02
72.0	3.78	4.06	4.02	3.98	3.95	3.91	3.87	3.84	3.80	3.76	3.73	3.69	3.66	3.62	3.58	3.55	3.51	3.47	3.44	3.40	3.36	3.33	3.29	3.25	3.22	3.18	3.15
73.0	3.91	4.18	4.15	4.11	4.07	4.04	4.00	3.97	3.93	3.89	3.86	3.82	3.78	3.75	3.71	3.67	3.64	3.60	3.56	3.53	3.49	3.46	3.42	3.38	3.35	3.31	3.27
74.0	4.04	4.31	4.28	4.24	4.20	4.17	4.13	4.10	4.06	4.02	3.99	3.95	3.91	3.88	3.84	3.80	3.77	3.73	3.69	3.66	3.62	3.59	3.55	3.51	3.48	3.44	3.40
75.0	4.17	4.44	4.41	4.37	4.34	4.30	4.26	4.23	4.19	4.15	4.12	4.08	4.04	4.01	3.97	3.94	3.90	3.86	3.83	3.79	3.75	3.72	3.68	3.64	3.61	3.57	3.53
76.0	4.30	4.58	4.54	4.51	4.47	4.43	4.40	4.36	4.32	4.29	4.25	4.21	4.18	4.14	4.10	4.07	4.03	4.00	3.96	3.92	3.89	3.85	3.81	3.78	3.74	3.70	3.67
77.0	4.44	4.71	4.68	4.64	4.60	4.57	4.53	4.49	4.46	4.42	4.39	4.35	4.31	4.28	4.24	4.20	4.17	4.13	4.09	4.06	4.02	3.98	3.95	3.91	3.88	3.84	3.80
78.0	4.57	4.85	4.81	4.78	4.74	4.70	4.67	4.63	4.59	4.56	4.52	4.49	4.45	4.41	4.38	4.34	4.30	4.27	4.23	4.19	4.16	4.12	4.08	4.05	4.01	3.98	3.94
79.0	4.71	4.99	4.95	4.92	4.88	4.84	4.81	4.77	4.73	4.70	4.66	4.62	4.59	4.55	4.51	4.48	4.44	4.41	4.37	4.33	4.30	4.26	4.22	4.19	4.15	4.11	4.08

Predicted FEV$_1$ (L) - African American Males - NHANES III

Height (Inches)	18	20	22	24	26	28	30	32	34	36	38	40	42	44	46	48	50	52	54	56	58	60	62	64	66	68	70
60.0	2.73	2.94	2.90	2.85	2.81	2.76	2.71	2.67	2.62	2.57	2.53	2.48	2.44	2.39	2.34	2.30	2.25	2.20	2.16	2.11	2.07	2.02	1.97	1.93	1.88	1.84	1.79
61.0	2.83	3.05	3.00	2.95	2.91	2.86	2.82	2.77	2.72	2.68	2.63	2.58	2.54	2.49	2.45	2.40	2.35	2.31	2.26	2.22	2.17	2.12	2.08	2.03	1.98	1.94	1.89
62.0	2.94	3.15	3.11	3.06	3.01	2.97	2.92	2.87	2.83	2.78	2.74	2.69	2.64	2.60	2.55	2.50	2.46	2.41	2.37	2.32	2.27	2.23	2.18	2.14	2.09	2.04	2.00
63.0	3.04	3.26	3.21	3.17	3.12	3.07	3.03	2.98	2.93	2.89	2.84	2.80	2.75	2.70	2.66	2.61	2.57	2.52	2.47	2.43	2.38	2.33	2.29	2.24	2.20	2.15	2.10
64.0	3.15	3.37	3.32	3.27	3.23	3.18	3.14	3.09	3.04	3.00	2.95	2.90	2.86	2.81	2.77	2.72	2.67	2.63	2.58	2.53	2.49	2.44	2.40	2.35	2.30	2.26	2.21
65.0	3.26	3.48	3.43	3.38	3.34	3.29	3.24	3.20	3.15	3.11	3.06	3.01	2.97	2.92	2.88	2.83	2.78	2.74	2.69	2.64	2.60	2.55	2.51	2.46	2.41	2.37	2.32
66.0	3.37	3.59	3.54	3.49	3.45	3.40	3.36	3.31	3.26	3.22	3.17	3.13	3.08	3.03	2.99	2.94	2.89	2.85	2.80	2.76	2.71	2.66	2.62	2.57	2.53	2.48	2.43
67.0	3.49	3.70	3.65	3.61	3.56	3.52	3.47	3.42	3.38	3.33	3.28	3.24	3.19	3.15	3.10	3.05	3.01	2.96	2.92	2.87	2.82	2.78	2.73	2.68	2.64	2.59	2.55
68.0	3.60	3.82	3.77	3.72	3.68	3.63	3.58	3.54	3.49	3.45	3.40	3.35	3.31	3.26	3.22	3.17	3.12	3.08	3.03	2.98	2.94	2.89	2.85	2.80	2.75	2.71	2.66
69.0	3.72	3.93	3.89	3.84	3.79	3.75	3.70	3.65	3.61	3.56	3.52	3.47	3.42	3.38	3.33	3.29	3.24	3.19	3.15	3.10	3.05	3.01	2.96	2.92	2.87	2.82	2.78
70.0	3.84	4.05	4.00	3.96	3.91	3.87	3.82	3.77	3.73	3.68	3.63	3.59	3.54	3.50	3.45	3.40	3.36	3.31	3.27	3.22	3.17	3.13	3.08	3.03	2.99	2.94	2.90
71.0	3.96	4.17	4.12	4.08	4.03	3.99	3.94	3.89	3.85	3.80	3.75	3.71	3.66	3.62	3.57	3.52	3.48	3.43	3.39	3.34	3.29	3.25	3.20	3.15	3.11	3.06	3.02
72.0	4.08	4.29	4.25	4.20	4.15	4.11	4.06	4.01	3.97	3.92	3.88	3.83	3.78	3.74	3.69	3.65	3.60	3.55	3.51	3.46	3.41	3.37	3.32	3.28	3.23	3.18	3.14
73.0	4.20	4.42	4.37	4.32	4.28	4.23	4.18	4.14	4.09	4.05	4.00	3.95	3.91	3.86	3.82	3.77	3.72	3.68	3.63	3.58	3.54	3.49	3.45	3.40	3.35	3.31	3.26
74.0	4.33	4.54	4.49	4.45	4.40	4.36	4.31	4.26	4.22	4.17	4.12	4.08	4.03	3.99	3.94	3.89	3.85	3.80	3.76	3.71	3.66	3.62	3.57	3.52	3.48	3.43	3.39
75.0	4.45	4.67	4.62	4.58	4.53	4.48	4.44	4.39	4.34	4.30	4.25	4.21	4.16	4.11	4.07	4.02	3.97	3.93	3.88	3.84	3.79	3.74	3.70	3.65	3.61	3.56	3.51
76.0	4.58	4.80	4.75	4.70	4.66	4.61	4.57	4.52	4.47	4.43	4.38	4.33	4.29	4.24	4.20	4.15	4.10	4.06	4.01	3.96	3.92	3.87	3.83	3.78	3.73	3.69	3.64
77.0	4.71	4.93	4.88	4.83	4.79	4.74	4.70	4.65	4.60	4.56	4.51	4.46	4.42	4.37	4.33	4.28	4.23	4.19	4.14	4.09	4.05	4.00	3.96	3.91	3.86	3.82	3.77
78.0	4.84	5.06	5.01	4.97	4.92	4.87	4.83	4.78	4.73	4.69	4.64	4.60	4.55	4.50	4.46	4.41	4.37	4.32	4.27	4.23	4.18	4.13	4.09	4.04	4.00	3.95	3.90
79.0	4.98	5.19	5.15	5.10	5.05	5.01	4.96	4.91	4.87	4.82	4.78	4.73	4.68	4.64	4.59	4.55	4.50	4.45	4.41	4.36	4.31	4.27	4.22	4.18	4.13	4.08	4.04

LLN for FEV$_1$ (L) - African American Males - NHANES III

Height (Inches)	18	20	22	24	26	28	30	32	34	36	38	40	42	44	46	48	50	52	54	56	58	60	62	64	66	68	70
60.0	2.12	2.33	2.29	2.24	2.19	2.15	2.10	2.06	2.01	1.96	1.92	1.87	1.82	1.78	1.73	1.69	1.64	1.59	1.55	1.50	1.45	1.41	1.36	1.32	1.27	1.22	1.18
61.0	2.20	2.41	2.37	2.32	2.28	2.23	2.18	2.14	2.09	2.05	2.00	1.95	1.91	1.86	1.81	1.77	1.72	1.68	1.63	1.58	1.54	1.49	1.44	1.40	1.35	1.31	1.26
62.0	2.28	2.50	2.45	2.41	2.36	2.31	2.27	2.22	2.18	2.13	2.08	2.04	1.99	1.94	1.90	1.85	1.81	1.76	1.71	1.67	1.62	1.57	1.53	1.48	1.44	1.39	1.34
63.0	2.37	2.58	2.54	2.49	2.45	2.40	2.35	2.31	2.26	2.21	2.17	2.12	2.08	2.03	1.98	1.94	1.89	1.84	1.80	1.75	1.71	1.66	1.61	1.57	1.52	1.48	1.43
64.0	2.46	2.67	2.62	2.58	2.53	2.49	2.44	2.39	2.35	2.30	2.25	2.21	2.16	2.12	2.07	2.02	1.98	1.93	1.89	1.84	1.79	1.75	1.70	1.65	1.61	1.56	1.52
65.0	2.54	2.76	2.71	2.67	2.62	2.57	2.53	2.48	2.43	2.39	2.34	2.30	2.25	2.20	2.16	2.11	2.07	2.02	1.97	1.93	1.88	1.83	1.79	1.74	1.70	1.65	1.60
66.0	2.63	2.85	2.80	2.75	2.71	2.66	2.62	2.57	2.52	2.48	2.43	2.39	2.34	2.29	2.25	2.20	2.15	2.11	2.06	2.02	1.97	1.92	1.88	1.83	1.79	1.74	1.69
67.0	2.72	2.94	2.89	2.85	2.80	2.75	2.71	2.66	2.61	2.57	2.52	2.48	2.43	2.38	2.34	2.29	2.25	2.20	2.15	2.11	2.06	2.01	1.97	1.92	1.88	1.83	1.78
68.0	2.82	3.03	2.98	2.94	2.89	2.85	2.80	2.75	2.71	2.66	2.61	2.57	2.52	2.48	2.43	2.38	2.34	2.29	2.24	2.20	2.15	2.11	2.06	2.01	1.97	1.92	1.88
69.0	2.91	3.12	3.08	3.03	2.98	2.94	2.89	2.85	2.80	2.75	2.71	2.66	2.62	2.57	2.52	2.48	2.43	2.38	2.34	2.29	2.25	2.20	2.15	2.11	2.06	2.01	1.97
70.0	3.00	3.22	3.17	3.13	3.08	3.03	2.99	2.94	2.89	2.85	2.80	2.76	2.71	2.66	2.62	2.57	2.53	2.48	2.43	2.39	2.34	2.29	2.25	2.20	2.16	2.11	2.06
71.0	3.10	3.31	3.27	3.22	3.18	3.13	3.08	3.04	2.99	2.94	2.90	2.85	2.81	2.76	2.71	2.67	2.62	2.58	2.53	2.48	2.44	2.39	2.34	2.30	2.25	2.21	2.16
72.0	3.20	3.41	3.37	3.32	3.27	3.23	3.18	3.13	3.09	3.04	3.00	2.95	2.90	2.86	2.81	2.76	2.72	2.67	2.63	2.58	2.53	2.49	2.44	2.40	2.35	2.30	2.26
73.0	3.30	3.51	3.46	3.42	3.37	3.33	3.28	3.23	3.19	3.14	3.09	3.05	3.00	2.96	2.91	2.86	2.82	2.77	2.73	2.68	2.63	2.59	2.54	2.49	2.45	2.40	2.36
74.0	3.40	3.61	3.56	3.52	3.47	3.43	3.38	3.33	3.29	3.24	3.19	3.15	3.10	3.06	3.01	2.96	2.92	2.87	2.83	2.78	2.73	2.69	2.64	2.59	2.55	2.50	2.46
75.0	3.50	3.71	3.67	3.62	3.57	3.53	3.48	3.43	3.39	3.34	3.30	3.25	3.20	3.16	3.11	3.07	3.02	2.97	2.93	2.88	2.83	2.79	2.74	2.70	2.65	2.60	2.56
76.0	3.60	3.81	3.77	3.72	3.68	3.63	3.58	3.54	3.49	3.45	3.40	3.35	3.31	3.26	3.21	3.17	3.12	3.08	3.03	2.98	2.94	2.89	2.85	2.80	2.75	2.71	2.66
77.0	3.71	3.92	3.87	3.83	3.78	3.73	3.69	3.64	3.60	3.55	3.50	3.46	3.41	3.36	3.32	3.27	3.23	3.18	3.13	3.09	3.04	3.00	2.95	2.90	2.86	2.81	2.76
78.0	3.81	4.02	3.98	3.93	3.89	3.84	3.79	3.75	3.70	3.66	3.61	3.56	3.52	3.47	3.42	3.38	3.33	3.29	3.24	3.19	3.15	3.10	3.05	3.01	2.96	2.92	2.87
79.0	3.92	4.13	4.09	4.04	3.99	3.95	3.90	3.85	3.81	3.76	3.72	3.67	3.62	3.58	3.53	3.49	3.44	3.39	3.35	3.30	3.25	3.21	3.16	3.12	3.07	3.02	2.98

Predicted FVC (L) - Mexican American Males - NHANES III

Height (Inches)	Age																										
	18	20	22	24	26	28	30	32	34	36	38	40	42	44	46	48	50	52	54	56	58	60	62	64	66	68	70
56.0	3.28	3.59	3.56	3.52	3.49	3.45	3.41	3.37	3.33	3.29	3.24	3.20	3.15	3.10	3.05	3.00	2.94	2.89	2.83	2.77	2.71	2.65	2.59	2.53	2.46	2.40	2.33
57.0	3.41	3.72	3.69	3.65	3.62	3.58	3.54	3.50	3.46	3.42	3.37	3.33	3.28	3.23	3.18	3.13	3.07	3.02	2.96	2.90	2.84	2.78	2.72	2.66	2.59	2.53	2.46
58.0	3.54	3.85	3.82	3.79	3.75	3.71	3.67	3.63	3.59	3.55	3.50	3.46	3.41	3.36	3.31	3.26	3.21	3.15	3.09	3.04	2.98	2.92	2.85	2.79	2.72	2.66	2.59
59.0	3.68	3.99	3.96	3.92	3.89	3.85	3.81	3.77	3.73	3.68	3.64	3.59	3.55	3.50	3.45	3.39	3.34	3.28	3.23	3.17	3.11	3.05	2.99	2.92	2.86	2.79	2.72
60.0	3.81	4.13	4.09	4.06	4.02	3.98	3.95	3.91	3.86	3.82	3.78	3.73	3.68	3.63	3.58	3.53	3.48	3.42	3.37	3.31	3.25	3.19	3.13	3.06	3.00	2.93	2.86
61.0	3.95	4.27	4.23	4.20	4.16	4.12	4.09	4.04	4.00	3.96	3.91	3.87	3.82	3.77	3.72	3.67	3.62	3.56	3.50	3.45	3.39	3.33	3.26	3.20	3.14	3.07	3.00
62.0	4.09	4.41	4.37	4.34	4.30	4.27	4.23	4.19	4.14	4.10	4.06	4.01	3.96	3.91	3.86	3.81	3.76	3.70	3.65	3.59	3.53	3.47	3.41	3.34	3.28	3.21	3.14
63.0	4.24	4.55	4.52	4.48	4.45	4.41	4.37	4.33	4.29	4.24	4.20	4.15	4.11	4.06	4.01	3.95	3.90	3.85	3.79	3.73	3.67	3.61	3.55	3.49	3.42	3.35	3.29
64.0	4.38	4.70	4.66	4.63	4.59	4.56	4.52	4.48	4.43	4.39	4.35	4.30	4.25	4.20	4.15	4.10	4.05	3.99	3.94	3.88	3.82	3.76	3.70	3.63	3.57	3.50	3.43
65.0	4.53	4.84	4.81	4.78	4.74	4.70	4.66	4.62	4.58	4.54	4.49	4.45	4.40	4.35	4.30	4.25	4.20	4.14	4.08	4.03	3.97	3.91	3.84	3.78	3.71	3.65	3.58
66.0	4.68	5.00	4.96	4.93	4.89	4.85	4.82	4.77	4.73	4.69	4.65	4.60	4.55	4.50	4.45	4.40	4.35	4.29	4.23	4.18	4.12	4.06	3.99	3.93	3.87	3.80	3.73
67.0	4.84	5.15	5.12	5.08	5.04	5.01	4.97	4.93	4.89	4.84	4.80	4.75	4.70	4.65	4.60	4.55	4.50	4.44	4.39	4.33	4.27	4.21	4.15	4.08	4.02	3.95	3.88
68.0	4.99	5.30	5.27	5.24	5.20	5.16	5.12	5.08	5.04	5.00	4.95	4.91	4.86	4.81	4.76	4.71	4.65	4.60	4.54	4.48	4.43	4.36	4.30	4.24	4.17	4.11	4.04
69.0	5.15	5.46	5.43	5.39	5.36	5.32	5.28	5.24	5.20	5.16	5.11	5.06	5.02	4.97	4.92	4.87	4.81	4.76	4.70	4.64	4.58	4.52	4.46	4.40	4.33	4.26	4.20
70.0	5.31	5.62	5.59	5.55	5.52	5.48	5.44	5.40	5.36	5.32	5.27	5.22	5.18	5.13	5.08	5.02	4.97	4.92	4.86	4.80	4.74	4.68	4.62	4.56	4.49	4.42	4.36
71.0	5.47	5.78	5.75	5.72	5.68	5.64	5.60	5.56	5.52	5.48	5.43	5.39	5.34	5.29	5.24	5.19	5.13	5.08	5.02	4.96	4.91	4.84	4.78	4.72	4.65	4.59	4.52
72.0	5.63	5.95	5.91	5.88	5.84	5.81	5.77	5.73	5.69	5.64	5.60	5.55	5.50	5.45	5.40	5.35	5.30	5.24	5.19	5.13	5.07	5.01	4.95	4.88	4.82	4.75	4.68
73.0	5.80	6.11	6.08	6.05	6.01	5.97	5.93	5.89	5.85	5.81	5.76	5.72	5.67	5.62	5.57	5.52	5.46	5.41	5.35	5.30	5.24	5.18	5.11	5.05	4.98	4.92	4.85
74.0	5.97	6.28	6.25	6.22	6.18	6.14	6.10	6.06	6.02	5.98	5.93	5.89	5.84	5.79	5.74	5.69	5.63	5.58	5.52	5.46	5.41	5.34	5.28	5.22	5.15	5.09	5.02
75.0	6.14	6.45	6.42	6.39	6.35	6.31	6.27	6.23	6.19	6.15	6.10	6.06	6.01	5.96	5.91	5.86	5.81	5.75	5.69	5.64	5.58	5.52	5.45	5.39	5.32	5.26	5.19
76.0	6.32	6.63	6.60	6.56	6.52	6.49	6.45	6.41	6.37	6.32	6.28	6.23	6.18	6.13	6.08	6.03	5.98	5.92	5.87	5.81	5.75	5.69	5.63	5.56	5.50	5.43	5.36
77.0	6.49	6.80	6.77	6.74	6.70	6.66	6.62	6.58	6.54	6.50	6.45	6.41	6.36	6.31	6.26	6.21	6.15	6.10	6.04	5.99	5.93	5.87	5.80	5.74	5.67	5.61	5.54
78.0	6.67	6.98	6.95	6.91	6.88	6.84	6.80	6.76	6.72	6.68	6.63	6.59	6.54	6.49	6.44	6.39	6.33	6.28	6.22	6.16	6.10	6.04	5.98	5.92	5.85	5.79	5.72

LLN for FVC (L) - Mexican American Males - NHANES III

Height (Inches)	Age																										
	18	20	22	24	26	28	30	32	34	36	38	40	42	44	46	48	50	52	54	56	58	60	62	64	66	68	70
56.0	2.70	3.01	2.98	2.94	2.91	2.87	2.83	2.79	2.75	2.71	2.66	2.61	2.57	2.52	2.47	2.41	2.36	2.31	2.25	2.19	2.13	2.07	2.01	1.95	1.88	1.81	1.75
57.0	2.81	3.12	3.09	3.05	3.02	2.98	2.94	2.90	2.86	2.81	2.77	2.72	2.68	2.63	2.58	2.52	2.47	2.42	2.36	2.30	2.24	2.18	2.12	2.05	1.99	1.92	1.86
58.0	2.92	3.23	3.20	3.16	3.13	3.09	3.05	3.01	2.97	2.92	2.88	2.83	2.79	2.74	2.69	2.63	2.58	2.53	2.47	2.41	2.35	2.29	2.23	2.17	2.10	2.03	1.97
59.0	3.03	3.34	3.31	3.28	3.24	3.20	3.16	3.12	3.08	3.04	2.99	2.95	2.90	2.85	2.80	2.75	2.69	2.64	2.58	2.52	2.47	2.40	2.34	2.28	2.21	2.15	2.08
60.0	3.15	3.46	3.43	3.39	3.35	3.32	3.28	3.24	3.20	3.15	3.11	3.06	3.01	2.96	2.91	2.86	2.81	2.75	2.70	2.64	2.58	2.52	2.46	2.39	2.33	2.26	2.19
61.0	3.26	3.57	3.54	3.51	3.47	3.43	3.39	3.35	3.31	3.27	3.22	3.18	3.13	3.08	3.03	2.98	2.93	2.87	2.81	2.76	2.70	2.64	2.57	2.51	2.44	2.38	2.31
62.0	3.38	3.69	3.66	3.63	3.59	3.55	3.51	3.47	3.43	3.39	3.34	3.30	3.25	3.20	3.15	3.10	3.04	2.99	2.93	2.87	2.82	2.75	2.69	2.63	2.56	2.50	2.43
63.0	3.50	3.81	3.78	3.75	3.71	3.67	3.63	3.59	3.55	3.51	3.46	3.42	3.37	3.32	3.27	3.22	3.16	3.11	3.05	3.00	2.94	2.88	2.81	2.75	2.68	2.62	2.55
64.0	3.62	3.94	3.90	3.87	3.83	3.80	3.76	3.72	3.67	3.63	3.59	3.54	3.49	3.44	3.39	3.34	3.29	3.23	3.18	3.12	3.06	3.00	2.94	2.87	2.81	2.74	2.67
65.0	3.75	4.06	4.03	3.99	3.96	3.92	3.88	3.84	3.80	3.76	3.71	3.66	3.62	3.57	3.52	3.46	3.41	3.36	3.30	3.24	3.18	3.12	3.06	3.00	2.93	2.86	2.80
66.0	3.87	4.19	4.15	4.12	4.08	4.05	4.01	3.97	3.92	3.88	3.84	3.79	3.74	3.69	3.64	3.59	3.54	3.48	3.43	3.37	3.31	3.25	3.19	3.12	3.06	2.99	2.92
67.0	4.00	4.32	4.28	4.25	4.21	4.17	4.14	4.09	4.05	4.01	3.97	3.92	3.87	3.82	3.77	3.72	3.67	3.61	3.55	3.50	3.44	3.38	3.31	3.25	3.19	3.12	3.05
68.0	4.13	4.45	4.41	4.38	4.34	4.30	4.27	4.23	4.18	4.14	4.10	4.05	4.00	3.95	3.90	3.85	3.80	3.74	3.68	3.63	3.57	3.51	3.44	3.38	3.32	3.25	3.18
69.0	4.26	4.58	4.54	4.51	4.47	4.44	4.40	4.36	4.32	4.27	4.23	4.18	4.13	4.08	4.03	3.98	3.93	3.87	3.82	3.76	3.70	3.64	3.58	3.51	3.45	3.38	3.31
70.0	4.40	4.71	4.68	4.64	4.61	4.57	4.53	4.49	4.45	4.41	4.36	4.32	4.27	4.22	4.17	4.12	4.06	4.01	3.95	3.89	3.83	3.77	3.71	3.65	3.58	3.52	3.45
71.0	4.53	4.85	4.81	4.78	4.74	4.71	4.67	4.63	4.59	4.54	4.50	4.45	4.40	4.35	4.30	4.25	4.20	4.14	4.09	4.03	3.97	3.91	3.85	3.78	3.72	3.65	3.58
72.0	4.67	4.99	4.95	4.92	4.88	4.84	4.81	4.77	4.72	4.68	4.64	4.59	4.54	4.49	4.44	4.39	4.34	4.28	4.22	4.17	4.11	4.05	3.98	3.92	3.86	3.79	3.72
73.0	4.81	5.13	5.09	5.06	5.02	4.98	4.95	4.90	4.86	4.82	4.78	4.73	4.68	4.63	4.58	4.53	4.48	4.42	4.36	4.31	4.25	4.19	4.12	4.06	4.00	3.93	3.86
74.0	4.95	5.27	5.23	5.20	5.16	5.13	5.09	5.05	5.00	4.96	4.92	4.87	4.82	4.77	4.72	4.67	4.62	4.56	4.51	4.45	4.39	4.33	4.27	4.20	4.14	4.07	4.00
75.0	5.10	5.41	5.38	5.34	5.31	5.27	5.23	5.19	5.15	5.11	5.06	5.01	4.97	4.92	4.87	4.81	4.76	4.71	4.65	4.59	4.53	4.47	4.41	4.35	4.28	4.21	4.15
76.0	5.24	5.56	5.52	5.49	5.45	5.42	5.38	5.34	5.29	5.25	5.21	5.16	5.11	5.06	5.01	4.96	4.91	4.85	4.80	4.74	4.68	4.62	4.56	4.49	4.43	4.36	4.29
77.0	5.39	5.70	5.67	5.64	5.60	5.56	5.52	5.48	5.44	5.40	5.35	5.31	5.26	5.21	5.16	5.11	5.05	5.00	4.94	4.89	4.83	4.77	4.70	4.64	4.57	4.51	4.44
78.0	5.54	5.85	5.82	5.79	5.75	5.71	5.67	5.63	5.59	5.55	5.50	5.46	5.41	5.36	5.31	5.26	5.20	5.15	5.09	5.03	4.98	4.91	4.85	4.79	4.72	4.66	4.59

Predicted FEV$_1$ (L) - Mexican American Males - NHANES III

Height (Inches)	18	20	22	24	26	28	30	32	34	36	38	40	42	44	46	48	50	52	54	56	58	60	62	64	66	68	70
56.0	2.86	3.10	3.04	2.98	2.93	2.87	2.81	2.75	2.69	2.63	2.57	2.52	2.46	2.40	2.34	2.28	2.22	2.16	2.11	2.05	1.99	1.93	1.87	1.81	1.75	1.70	1.64
57.0	2.97	3.21	3.15	3.09	3.04	2.98	2.92	2.86	2.80	2.74	2.68	2.63	2.57	2.51	2.45	2.39	2.33	2.27	2.22	2.16	2.10	2.04	1.98	1.92	1.86	1.81	1.75
58.0	3.08	3.32	3.26	3.21	3.15	3.09	3.03	2.97	2.91	2.85	2.80	2.74	2.68	2.62	2.56	2.50	2.44	2.39	2.33	2.27	2.21	2.15	2.09	2.03	1.98	1.92	1.86
59.0	3.20	3.44	3.38	3.32	3.26	3.20	3.14	3.09	3.03	2.97	2.91	2.85	2.79	2.73	2.68	2.62	2.56	2.50	2.44	2.38	2.32	2.27	2.21	2.15	2.09	2.03	1.97
60.0	3.31	3.55	3.49	3.44	3.38	3.32	3.26	3.20	3.14	3.08	3.03	2.97	2.91	2.85	2.79	2.73	2.67	2.62	2.56	2.50	2.44	2.38	2.32	2.26	2.21	2.15	2.09
61.0	3.43	3.67	3.61	3.55	3.50	3.44	3.38	3.32	3.26	3.20	3.14	3.09	3.03	2.97	2.91	2.85	2.79	2.73	2.68	2.62	2.56	2.50	2.44	2.38	2.32	2.27	2.21
62.0	3.55	3.79	3.73	3.67	3.62	3.56	3.50	3.44	3.38	3.32	3.26	3.21	3.15	3.09	3.03	2.97	2.91	2.85	2.80	2.74	2.68	2.62	2.56	2.50	2.44	2.39	2.33
63.0	3.67	3.91	3.85	3.80	3.74	3.68	3.62	3.56	3.50	3.44	3.39	3.33	3.27	3.21	3.15	3.09	3.03	2.98	2.92	2.86	2.80	2.74	2.68	2.62	2.57	2.51	2.45
64.0	3.80	4.04	3.98	3.92	3.86	3.80	3.74	3.68	3.63	3.57	3.51	3.45	3.39	3.33	3.28	3.22	3.16	3.10	3.04	2.98	2.92	2.87	2.81	2.75	2.69	2.63	2.57
65.0	3.92	4.16	4.10	4.04	3.99	3.93	3.87	3.81	3.75	3.69	3.64	3.58	3.52	3.46	3.40	3.34	3.28	3.23	3.17	3.11	3.05	2.99	2.93	2.87	2.82	2.76	2.70
66.0	4.05	4.29	4.23	4.17	4.11	4.06	4.00	3.94	3.88	3.82	3.76	3.70	3.65	3.59	3.53	3.47	3.41	3.35	3.29	3.24	3.18	3.12	3.06	3.00	2.94	2.88	2.83
67.0	4.18	4.42	4.36	4.30	4.24	4.19	4.13	4.07	4.01	3.95	3.89	3.83	3.78	3.72	3.66	3.60	3.54	3.48	3.42	3.37	3.31	3.25	3.19	3.13	3.07	3.01	2.96
68.0	4.31	4.55	4.49	4.43	4.38	4.32	4.26	4.20	4.14	4.08	4.02	3.97	3.91	3.85	3.79	3.73	3.67	3.61	3.56	3.50	3.44	3.38	3.32	3.26	3.20	3.15	3.09
69.0	4.44	4.68	4.63	4.57	4.51	4.45	4.39	4.33	4.27	4.22	4.16	4.10	4.04	3.98	3.92	3.86	3.81	3.75	3.69	3.63	3.57	3.51	3.45	3.40	3.34	3.28	3.22
70.0	4.58	4.82	4.76	4.70	4.64	4.59	4.53	4.47	4.41	4.35	4.29	4.23	4.18	4.12	4.06	4.00	3.94	3.88	3.82	3.77	3.71	3.65	3.59	3.53	3.47	3.41	3.36
71.0	4.72	4.96	4.90	4.84	4.78	4.72	4.66	4.61	4.55	4.49	4.43	4.37	4.31	4.25	4.20	4.14	4.08	4.02	3.96	3.90	3.84	3.79	3.73	3.67	3.61	3.55	3.49
72.0	4.86	5.10	5.04	4.98	4.92	4.86	4.80	4.75	4.69	4.63	4.57	4.51	4.45	4.39	4.34	4.28	4.22	4.16	4.10	4.04	3.98	3.93	3.87	3.81	3.75	3.69	3.63
73.0	5.00	5.24	5.18	5.12	5.06	5.00	4.95	4.89	4.83	4.77	4.71	4.65	4.59	4.54	4.48	4.42	4.36	4.30	4.24	4.18	4.13	4.07	4.01	3.95	3.89	3.83	3.77
74.0	5.14	5.38	5.32	5.26	5.21	5.15	5.09	5.03	4.97	4.91	4.85	4.80	4.74	4.68	4.62	4.56	4.50	4.44	4.39	4.33	4.27	4.21	4.15	4.09	4.03	3.98	3.92
75.0	5.29	5.53	5.47	5.41	5.35	5.29	5.23	5.17	5.12	5.06	5.00	4.94	4.88	4.82	4.76	4.71	4.65	4.59	4.53	4.47	4.41	4.36	4.30	4.24	4.18	4.12	4.06
76.0	5.43	5.67	5.61	5.56	5.50	5.44	5.38	5.32	5.26	5.20	5.15	5.09	5.03	4.97	4.91	4.85	4.80	4.74	4.68	4.62	4.56	4.50	4.44	4.39	4.33	4.27	4.21
77.0	5.58	5.82	5.76	5.71	5.65	5.59	5.53	5.47	5.41	5.35	5.30	5.24	5.18	5.12	5.06	5.00	4.94	4.89	4.83	4.77	4.71	4.65	4.59	4.53	4.48	4.42	4.36
78.0	5.73	5.97	5.91	5.86	5.80	5.74	5.68	5.62	5.56	5.51	5.45	5.39	5.33	5.27	5.21	5.15	5.10	5.04	4.98	4.92	4.86	4.80	4.74	4.69	4.63	4.57	4.51

LLN for FEV$_1$ (L) - Mexican American Males - NHANES III

Height (Inches)	18	20	22	24	26	28	30	32	34	36	38	40	42	44	46	48	50	52	54	56	58	60	62	64	66	68	70
56.0	2.37	2.61	2.55	2.49	2.43	2.37	2.32	2.26	2.20	2.14	2.08	2.02	1.96	1.91	1.85	1.79	1.73	1.67	1.61	1.55	1.50	1.44	1.38	1.32	1.26	1.20	1.14
57.0	2.46	2.70	2.64	2.58	2.53	2.47	2.41	2.35	2.29	2.23	2.17	2.12	2.06	2.00	1.94	1.88	1.82	1.76	1.71	1.65	1.59	1.53	1.47	1.41	1.35	1.30	1.24
58.0	2.55	2.79	2.74	2.68	2.62	2.56	2.50	2.44	2.38	2.33	2.27	2.21	2.15	2.09	2.03	1.97	1.92	1.86	1.80	1.74	1.68	1.62	1.57	1.51	1.45	1.39	1.33
59.0	2.65	2.89	2.83	2.77	2.71	2.66	2.60	2.54	2.48	2.42	2.36	2.30	2.25	2.19	2.13	2.07	2.01	1.95	1.89	1.84	1.78	1.72	1.66	1.60	1.54	1.48	1.43
60.0	2.75	2.99	2.93	2.87	2.81	2.75	2.69	2.64	2.58	2.52	2.46	2.40	2.34	2.28	2.23	2.17	2.11	2.05	1.99	1.93	1.88	1.82	1.76	1.70	1.64	1.58	1.52
61.0	2.85	3.09	3.03	2.97	2.91	2.85	2.79	2.74	2.68	2.62	2.56	2.50	2.44	2.38	2.33	2.27	2.21	2.15	2.09	2.03	1.97	1.92	1.86	1.80	1.74	1.68	1.62
62.0	2.95	3.19	3.13	3.07	3.01	2.95	2.89	2.84	2.78	2.72	2.66	2.60	2.54	2.48	2.43	2.37	2.31	2.25	2.19	2.13	2.07	2.02	1.96	1.90	1.84	1.78	1.72
63.0	3.05	3.29	3.23	3.17	3.11	3.06	3.00	2.94	2.88	2.82	2.76	2.70	2.65	2.59	2.53	2.47	2.41	2.35	2.29	2.24	2.18	2.12	2.06	2.00	1.94	1.88	1.83
64.0	3.15	3.39	3.33	3.28	3.22	3.16	3.10	3.04	2.98	2.92	2.87	2.81	2.75	2.69	2.63	2.57	2.51	2.46	2.40	2.34	2.28	2.22	2.16	2.10	2.05	1.99	1.93
65.0	3.26	3.50	3.44	3.38	3.32	3.26	3.21	3.15	3.09	3.03	2.97	2.91	2.85	2.80	2.74	2.68	2.62	2.56	2.50	2.44	2.39	2.33	2.27	2.21	2.15	2.09	2.03
66.0	3.36	3.61	3.55	3.49	3.43	3.37	3.31	3.25	3.20	3.14	3.08	3.02	2.96	2.90	2.84	2.79	2.73	2.67	2.61	2.55	2.49	2.43	2.38	2.32	2.26	2.20	2.14
67.0	3.47	3.71	3.66	3.60	3.54	3.48	3.42	3.36	3.30	3.25	3.19	3.13	3.07	3.01	2.95	2.89	2.84	2.78	2.72	2.66	2.60	2.54	2.48	2.43	2.37	2.31	2.25
68.0	3.58	3.82	3.77	3.71	3.65	3.59	3.53	3.47	3.41	3.36	3.30	3.24	3.18	3.12	3.06	3.00	2.95	2.89	2.83	2.77	2.71	2.65	2.59	2.54	2.48	2.42	2.36
69.0	3.70	3.94	3.88	3.82	3.76	3.70	3.64	3.59	3.53	3.47	3.41	3.35	3.29	3.23	3.18	3.12	3.06	3.00	2.94	2.88	2.82	2.77	2.71	2.65	2.59	2.53	2.47
70.0	3.81	4.05	3.99	3.93	3.87	3.82	3.76	3.70	3.64	3.58	3.52	3.46	3.41	3.35	3.29	3.23	3.17	3.11	3.05	3.00	2.94	2.88	2.82	2.76	2.70	2.64	2.59
71.0	3.92	4.17	4.11	4.05	3.99	3.93	3.87	3.81	3.76	3.70	3.64	3.58	3.52	3.46	3.40	3.35	3.29	3.23	3.17	3.11	3.05	2.99	2.94	2.88	2.82	2.76	2.70
72.0	4.04	4.28	4.22	4.17	4.11	4.05	3.99	3.93	3.87	3.81	3.76	3.70	3.64	3.58	3.52	3.46	3.40	3.35	3.29	3.23	3.17	3.11	3.05	2.99	2.94	2.88	2.82
73.0	4.16	4.40	4.34	4.28	4.23	4.17	4.11	4.05	3.99	3.93	3.87	3.82	3.76	3.70	3.64	3.58	3.52	3.46	3.41	3.35	3.29	3.23	3.17	3.11	3.05	3.00	2.94
74.0	4.28	4.52	4.46	4.40	4.35	4.29	4.23	4.17	4.11	4.05	3.99	3.94	3.88	3.82	3.76	3.70	3.64	3.58	3.53	3.47	3.41	3.35	3.29	3.23	3.17	3.12	3.06
75.0	4.40	4.64	4.58	4.53	4.47	4.41	4.35	4.29	4.23	4.17	4.12	4.06	4.00	3.94	3.88	3.82	3.76	3.71	3.65	3.59	3.53	3.47	3.41	3.35	3.30	3.24	3.18
76.0	4.53	4.77	4.71	4.65	4.59	4.53	4.47	4.42	4.36	4.30	4.24	4.18	4.12	4.06	4.01	3.95	3.89	3.83	3.77	3.71	3.65	3.60	3.54	3.48	3.42	3.36	3.30
77.0	4.65	4.89	4.83	4.77	4.72	4.66	4.60	4.54	4.48	4.42	4.36	4.31	4.25	4.19	4.13	4.07	4.01	3.95	3.90	3.84	3.78	3.72	3.66	3.60	3.54	3.49	3.43
78.0	4.78	5.02	4.96	4.90	4.84	4.78	4.73	4.67	4.61	4.55	4.49	4.43	4.37	4.32	4.26	4.20	4.14	4.08	4.02	3.96	3.91	3.85	3.79	3.73	3.67	3.61	3.55

Predicted FVC (L) - Caucasian Females - NHANES III

Height (Inches)	18	20	22	24	26	28	30	32	34	36	38	40	42	44	46	48	50	52	54	56	58	60	62	64	66	68	70
57.0	2.96	2.97	2.98	2.98	2.98	2.97	2.97	2.96	2.94	2.93	2.91	2.89	2.86	2.83	2.80	2.77	2.73	2.69	2.65	2.60	2.55	2.50	2.44	2.38	2.32	2.25	2.19
58.0	3.07	3.08	3.09	3.09	3.09	3.08	3.08	3.07	3.05	3.04	3.02	3.00	2.97	2.94	2.91	2.88	2.84	2.80	2.76	2.71	2.66	2.61	2.55	2.49	2.43	2.36	2.30
59.0	3.18	3.19	3.20	3.20	3.20	3.20	3.19	3.18	3.17	3.15	3.13	3.11	3.08	3.05	3.02	2.99	2.95	2.91	2.87	2.82	2.77	2.72	2.66	2.60	2.54	2.48	2.41
60.0	3.30	3.31	3.31	3.31	3.31	3.31	3.30	3.29	3.28	3.26	3.24	3.22	3.20	3.17	3.14	3.10	3.06	3.02	2.98	2.93	2.88	2.83	2.78	2.72	2.66	2.59	2.52
61.0	3.41	3.42	3.43	3.43	3.43	3.42	3.42	3.41	3.39	3.38	3.36	3.34	3.31	3.28	3.25	3.22	3.18	3.14	3.10	3.05	3.00	2.95	2.89	2.83	2.77	2.71	2.64
62.0	3.53	3.54	3.54	3.55	3.55	3.54	3.54	3.53	3.51	3.50	3.48	3.45	3.43	3.40	3.37	3.34	3.30	3.26	3.21	3.17	3.12	3.06	3.01	2.95	2.89	2.82	2.76
63.0	3.65	3.66	3.66	3.67	3.67	3.66	3.65	3.64	3.63	3.62	3.60	3.57	3.55	3.52	3.49	3.46	3.42	3.38	3.33	3.29	3.24	3.18	3.13	3.07	3.01	2.94	2.87
64.0	3.77	3.78	3.79	3.79	3.79	3.78	3.78	3.77	3.75	3.74	3.72	3.70	3.67	3.64	3.61	3.58	3.54	3.50	3.45	3.41	3.36	3.31	3.25	3.19	3.13	3.06	3.00
65.0	3.90	3.90	3.91	3.91	3.91	3.91	3.90	3.89	3.88	3.86	3.84	3.82	3.79	3.77	3.73	3.70	3.66	3.62	3.58	3.53	3.48	3.43	3.37	3.31	3.25	3.19	3.12
66.0	4.02	4.03	4.03	4.04	4.04	4.03	4.02	4.01	4.00	3.99	3.97	3.94	3.92	3.89	3.86	3.82	3.79	3.75	3.70	3.66	3.61	3.55	3.50	3.44	3.38	3.31	3.24
67.0	4.15	4.16	4.16	4.16	4.16	4.16	4.15	4.14	4.13	4.11	4.09	4.07	4.05	4.02	3.99	3.95	3.91	3.87	3.83	3.78	3.73	3.68	3.63	3.57	3.50	3.44	3.37
68.0	4.28	4.28	4.29	4.29	4.29	4.29	4.28	4.27	4.26	4.24	4.22	4.20	4.18	4.15	4.12	4.08	4.04	4.00	3.96	3.91	3.86	3.81	3.75	3.70	3.63	3.57	3.50
69.0	4.41	4.42	4.42	4.42	4.42	4.42	4.41	4.40	4.39	4.37	4.35	4.33	4.31	4.28	4.25	4.21	4.17	4.13	4.09	4.04	3.99	3.94	3.89	3.83	3.76	3.70	3.63
70.0	4.54	4.55	4.55	4.56	4.56	4.55	4.54	4.53	4.52	4.51	4.49	4.46	4.44	4.41	4.38	4.34	4.31	4.27	4.22	4.18	4.13	4.07	4.02	3.96	3.90	3.83	3.76
71.0	4.68	4.68	4.69	4.69	4.69	4.69	4.68	4.67	4.66	4.64	4.62	4.60	4.57	4.55	4.51	4.48	4.44	4.40	4.36	4.31	4.26	4.21	4.15	4.09	4.03	3.97	3.90
72.0	4.81	4.82	4.83	4.83	4.83	4.82	4.82	4.81	4.79	4.78	4.76	4.74	4.71	4.68	4.65	4.62	4.58	4.54	4.49	4.45	4.40	4.35	4.29	4.23	4.17	4.10	4.04
73.0	4.95	4.96	4.96	4.97	4.97	4.96	4.95	4.94	4.93	4.92	4.90	4.87	4.85	4.82	4.79	4.75	4.72	4.68	4.63	4.59	4.54	4.48	4.43	4.37	4.31	4.24	4.17
74.0	5.09	5.10	5.10	5.11	5.11	5.10	5.10	5.09	5.07	5.06	5.04	5.01	4.99	4.96	4.93	4.90	4.86	4.82	4.77	4.73	4.68	4.62	4.57	4.51	4.45	4.38	4.32

LLN for FVC (L) - Caucasian Females - NHANES III

Height (Inches)	18	20	22	24	26	28	30	32	34	36	38	40	42	44	46	48	50	52	54	56	58	60	62	64	66	68	70
57.0	2.41	2.42	2.43	2.43	2.43	2.42	2.42	2.41	2.40	2.38	2.36	2.34	2.31	2.28	2.25	2.22	2.18	2.14	2.10	2.05	2.00	1.95	1.89	1.83	1.77	1.71	1.64
58.0	2.50	2.51	2.52	2.52	2.52	2.52	2.51	2.50	2.49	2.47	2.45	2.43	2.40	2.37	2.34	2.31	2.27	2.23	2.19	2.14	2.09	2.04	1.98	1.92	1.86	1.80	1.73
59.0	2.60	2.60	2.61	2.61	2.61	2.61	2.60	2.59	2.58	2.56	2.54	2.52	2.49	2.47	2.44	2.40	2.36	2.32	2.28	2.23	2.18	2.13	2.07	2.02	1.95	1.89	1.82
60.0	2.69	2.70	2.70	2.71	2.71	2.70	2.69	2.68	2.67	2.66	2.64	2.61	2.59	2.56	2.53	2.49	2.46	2.42	2.37	2.33	2.28	2.22	2.17	2.11	2.05	1.98	1.91
61.0	2.79	2.79	2.80	2.80	2.80	2.80	2.79	2.78	2.77	2.75	2.73	2.71	2.68	2.66	2.62	2.59	2.55	2.51	2.47	2.42	2.37	2.32	2.26	2.20	2.14	2.08	2.01
62.0	2.88	2.89	2.90	2.90	2.90	2.89	2.89	2.88	2.86	2.85	2.83	2.81	2.78	2.75	2.72	2.69	2.65	2.61	2.56	2.52	2.47	2.42	2.36	2.30	2.24	2.17	2.11
63.0	2.98	2.99	2.99	3.00	3.00	2.99	2.98	2.97	2.96	2.95	2.93	2.90	2.88	2.85	2.82	2.78	2.75	2.71	2.66	2.62	2.57	2.51	2.46	2.40	2.34	2.27	2.20
64.0	3.08	3.09	3.09	3.10	3.10	3.09	3.08	3.07	3.06	3.05	3.03	3.00	2.98	2.95	2.92	2.88	2.85	2.81	2.76	2.72	2.67	2.61	2.56	2.50	2.44	2.37	2.30
65.0	3.18	3.19	3.20	3.20	3.20	3.19	3.19	3.18	3.16	3.15	3.13	3.11	3.08	3.05	3.02	2.99	2.95	2.91	2.86	2.82	2.77	2.72	2.66	2.60	2.54	2.47	2.41
66.0	3.28	3.29	3.30	3.30	3.30	3.30	3.29	3.28	3.27	3.25	3.23	3.21	3.18	3.16	3.12	3.09	3.05	3.01	2.97	2.92	2.87	2.82	2.76	2.70	2.64	2.58	2.51
67.0	3.39	3.40	3.40	3.41	3.40	3.40	3.39	3.38	3.37	3.35	3.34	3.31	3.29	3.26	3.23	3.19	3.16	3.12	3.07	3.03	2.98	2.92	2.87	2.81	2.75	2.68	2.61
68.0	3.50	3.50	3.51	3.51	3.51	3.51	3.50	3.49	3.48	3.46	3.44	3.42	3.39	3.37	3.33	3.30	3.26	3.22	3.18	3.13	3.08	3.03	2.97	2.92	2.85	2.79	2.72
69.0	3.60	3.61	3.62	3.62	3.62	3.61	3.61	3.60	3.58	3.57	3.55	3.53	3.50	3.47	3.44	3.41	3.37	3.33	3.29	3.24	3.19	3.14	3.08	3.02	2.96	2.90	2.83
70.0	3.71	3.72	3.73	3.73	3.73	3.72	3.72	3.71	3.69	3.68	3.66	3.64	3.61	3.58	3.55	3.52	3.48	3.44	3.40	3.35	3.30	3.25	3.19	3.13	3.07	3.01	2.94
71.0	3.82	3.83	3.84	3.84	3.84	3.84	3.83	3.82	3.81	3.79	3.77	3.75	3.72	3.69	3.66	3.63	3.59	3.55	3.51	3.46	3.41	3.36	3.30	3.24	3.18	3.12	3.05
72.0	3.94	3.94	3.95	3.95	3.95	3.95	3.94	3.93	3.92	3.90	3.88	3.86	3.84	3.81	3.78	3.74	3.70	3.66	3.62	3.57	3.52	3.47	3.41	3.36	3.29	3.23	3.16
73.0	4.05	4.06	4.06	4.07	4.07	4.06	4.05	4.04	4.03	4.02	4.00	3.97	3.95	3.92	3.89	3.86	3.82	3.78	3.73	3.69	3.64	3.58	3.53	3.47	3.41	3.34	3.27
74.0	4.17	4.17	4.18	4.18	4.18	4.18	4.17	4.16	4.15	4.13	4.11	4.09	4.06	4.04	4.01	3.97	3.93	3.89	3.85	3.80	3.75	3.70	3.64	3.59	3.52	3.46	3.39

Predicted FEV$_1$ (L) - Caucasian Females - NHANES III

Height (Inches)	18	20	22	24	26	28	30	32	34	36	38	40	42	44	46	48	50	52	54	56	58	60	62	64	66	68	70
57.0	2.72	2.69	2.67	2.64	2.62	2.59	2.56	2.53	2.50	2.46	2.43	2.39	2.35	2.31	2.27	2.22	2.18	2.13	2.08	2.03	1.98	1.93	1.87	1.82	1.76	1.70	1.64
58.0	2.80	2.78	2.75	2.73	2.70	2.68	2.65	2.61	2.58	2.55	2.51	2.47	2.43	2.39	2.35	2.31	2.26	2.22	2.17	2.12	2.07	2.01	1.96	1.90	1.84	1.79	1.72
59.0	2.89	2.87	2.84	2.82	2.79	2.76	2.73	2.70	2.67	2.63	2.60	2.56	2.52	2.48	2.44	2.39	2.35	2.30	2.25	2.20	2.15	2.10	2.05	1.99	1.93	1.87	1.81
60.0	2.98	2.95	2.93	2.90	2.88	2.85	2.82	2.79	2.76	2.72	2.69	2.65	2.61	2.57	2.53	2.48	2.44	2.39	2.34	2.29	2.24	2.19	2.13	2.08	2.02	1.96	1.90
61.0	3.07	3.04	3.02	2.99	2.97	2.94	2.91	2.88	2.85	2.81	2.78	2.74	2.70	2.66	2.62	2.57	2.53	2.48	2.43	2.38	2.33	2.28	2.22	2.17	2.11	2.05	1.99
62.0	3.16	3.13	3.11	3.09	3.06	3.03	3.00	2.97	2.94	2.90	2.87	2.83	2.79	2.75	2.71	2.66	2.62	2.57	2.52	2.47	2.42	2.37	2.31	2.26	2.20	2.14	2.08
63.0	3.25	3.23	3.20	3.18	3.15	3.12	3.09	3.06	3.03	3.00	2.96	2.92	2.88	2.84	2.80	2.76	2.71	2.66	2.62	2.57	2.52	2.46	2.41	2.35	2.29	2.23	2.17
64.0	3.34	3.32	3.30	3.27	3.25	3.22	3.19	3.16	3.12	3.09	3.05	3.02	2.98	2.94	2.89	2.85	2.81	2.76	2.71	2.66	2.61	2.56	2.50	2.45	2.39	2.33	2.27
65.0	3.44	3.42	3.39	3.37	3.34	3.31	3.28	3.25	3.22	3.19	3.15	3.11	3.07	3.03	2.99	2.95	2.90	2.85	2.81	2.76	2.70	2.65	2.60	2.54	2.48	2.42	2.36
66.0	3.54	3.51	3.49	3.47	3.44	3.41	3.38	3.35	3.32	3.28	3.25	3.21	3.17	3.13	3.09	3.04	3.00	2.95	2.90	2.85	2.80	2.75	2.69	2.64	2.58	2.52	2.46
67.0	3.63	3.61	3.59	3.56	3.54	3.51	3.48	3.45	3.42	3.38	3.35	3.31	3.27	3.23	3.19	3.14	3.10	3.05	3.00	2.95	2.90	2.85	2.79	2.74	2.68	2.62	2.56
68.0	3.73	3.71	3.69	3.66	3.64	3.61	3.58	3.55	3.52	3.48	3.45	3.41	3.37	3.33	3.29	3.24	3.20	3.15	3.10	3.05	3.00	2.95	2.89	2.84	2.78	2.72	2.66
69.0	3.84	3.81	3.79	3.77	3.74	3.71	3.68	3.65	3.62	3.58	3.55	3.51	3.47	3.43	3.39	3.34	3.30	3.25	3.20	3.15	3.10	3.05	2.99	2.94	2.88	2.82	2.76
70.0	3.94	3.92	3.89	3.87	3.84	3.81	3.78	3.75	3.72	3.69	3.65	3.61	3.57	3.53	3.49	3.45	3.40	3.36	3.31	3.26	3.21	3.15	3.10	3.04	2.98	2.92	2.86
71.0	4.04	4.02	4.00	3.97	3.95	3.92	3.89	3.86	3.83	3.79	3.75	3.72	3.68	3.64	3.60	3.55	3.51	3.46	3.41	3.36	3.31	3.26	3.20	3.15	3.09	3.03	2.97
72.0	4.15	4.13	4.10	4.08	4.05	4.02	4.00	3.96	3.93	3.90	3.86	3.82	3.78	3.74	3.70	3.66	3.61	3.57	3.52	3.47	3.42	3.36	3.31	3.25	3.19	3.14	3.07
73.0	4.26	4.24	4.21	4.19	4.16	4.13	4.10	4.07	4.04	4.00	3.97	3.93	3.89	3.85	3.81	3.77	3.72	3.67	3.63	3.58	3.52	3.47	3.42	3.36	3.30	3.24	3.18
74.0	4.37	4.34	4.32	4.30	4.27	4.24	4.21	4.18	4.15	4.11	4.08	4.04	4.00	3.96	3.92	3.87	3.83	3.78	3.73	3.68	3.63	3.58	3.53	3.47	3.41	3.35	3.29

LLN for FEV$_1$ (L) - Caucasian Females - NHANES III

Height (Inches)	18	20	22	24	26	28	30	32	34	36	38	40	42	44	46	48	50	52	54	56	58	60	62	64	66	68	70
57.0	2.25	2.23	2.21	2.18	2.15	2.13	2.10	2.06	2.03	2.00	1.96	1.92	1.89	1.84	1.80	1.76	1.71	1.67	1.62	1.57	1.52	1.46	1.41	1.35	1.30	1.24	1.18
58.0	2.32	2.30	2.27	2.25	2.22	2.19	2.17	2.13	2.10	2.07	2.03	1.99	1.95	1.91	1.87	1.83	1.78	1.74	1.69	1.64	1.59	1.53	1.48	1.42	1.36	1.31	1.24
59.0	2.39	2.37	2.34	2.32	2.29	2.26	2.24	2.20	2.17	2.14	2.10	2.06	2.02	1.98	1.94	1.90	1.85	1.81	1.76	1.71	1.66	1.60	1.55	1.49	1.43	1.38	1.31
60.0	2.46	2.44	2.42	2.39	2.36	2.34	2.31	2.28	2.24	2.21	2.17	2.13	2.10	2.05	2.01	1.97	1.92	1.88	1.83	1.78	1.73	1.67	1.62	1.56	1.51	1.45	1.39
61.0	2.53	2.51	2.49	2.46	2.44	2.41	2.38	2.35	2.31	2.28	2.24	2.21	2.17	2.13	2.09	2.04	2.00	1.95	1.90	1.85	1.80	1.75	1.69	1.64	1.58	1.52	1.46
62.0	2.61	2.59	2.56	2.54	2.51	2.48	2.45	2.42	2.39	2.35	2.32	2.28	2.24	2.20	2.16	2.12	2.07	2.02	1.97	1.92	1.87	1.82	1.77	1.71	1.65	1.59	1.53
63.0	2.68	2.66	2.64	2.61	2.59	2.56	2.53	2.50	2.46	2.43	2.39	2.36	2.32	2.28	2.23	2.19	2.14	2.10	2.05	2.00	1.95	1.90	1.84	1.78	1.73	1.67	1.61
64.0	2.76	2.74	2.71	2.69	2.66	2.63	2.60	2.57	2.54	2.51	2.47	2.43	2.39	2.35	2.31	2.27	2.22	2.17	2.13	2.08	2.02	1.97	1.92	1.86	1.80	1.74	1.68
65.0	2.84	2.81	2.79	2.77	2.74	2.71	2.68	2.65	2.62	2.58	2.55	2.51	2.47	2.43	2.39	2.34	2.30	2.25	2.20	2.15	2.10	2.05	1.99	1.94	1.88	1.82	1.76
66.0	2.91	2.89	2.87	2.84	2.82	2.79	2.76	2.73	2.70	2.66	2.62	2.59	2.55	2.51	2.47	2.42	2.38	2.33	2.28	2.23	2.18	2.13	2.07	2.02	1.96	1.90	1.84
67.0	2.99	2.97	2.95	2.92	2.90	2.87	2.84	2.81	2.77	2.74	2.70	2.67	2.63	2.59	2.55	2.50	2.46	2.41	2.36	2.31	2.26	2.21	2.15	2.10	2.04	1.98	1.92
68.0	3.07	3.05	3.03	3.00	2.98	2.95	2.92	2.89	2.86	2.82	2.79	2.75	2.71	2.67	2.63	2.58	2.54	2.49	2.44	2.39	2.34	2.29	2.23	2.18	2.12	2.06	2.00
69.0	3.16	3.13	3.11	3.09	3.06	3.03	3.00	2.97	2.94	2.90	2.87	2.83	2.79	2.75	2.71	2.66	2.62	2.57	2.52	2.47	2.42	2.37	2.32	2.26	2.20	2.14	2.08
70.0	3.24	3.22	3.19	3.17	3.14	3.11	3.09	3.05	3.02	2.99	2.95	2.91	2.87	2.83	2.79	2.75	2.70	2.66	2.61	2.56	2.51	2.45	2.40	2.34	2.28	2.23	2.16
71.0	3.32	3.30	3.28	3.25	3.23	3.20	3.17	3.14	3.11	3.07	3.04	3.00	2.96	2.92	2.88	2.83	2.79	2.74	2.69	2.64	2.59	2.54	2.48	2.43	2.37	2.31	2.25
72.0	3.41	3.39	3.36	3.34	3.31	3.28	3.26	3.22	3.19	3.16	3.12	3.08	3.04	3.00	2.96	2.92	2.87	2.83	2.78	2.73	2.68	2.62	2.57	2.51	2.45	2.40	2.33
73.0	3.50	3.48	3.45	3.43	3.40	3.37	3.34	3.31	3.28	3.24	3.21	3.17	3.13	3.09	3.05	3.00	2.96	2.91	2.86	2.81	2.76	2.71	2.66	2.60	2.54	2.48	2.42
74.0	3.59	3.56	3.54	3.51	3.49	3.46	3.43	3.40	3.37	3.33	3.30	3.26	3.22	3.18	3.14	3.09	3.05	3.00	2.95	2.90	2.85	2.80	2.74	2.69	2.63	2.57	2.51

Predicted FVC (L) - African American Females - NHANES III

Height (Inches)	18	20	22	24	26	28	30	32	34	36	38	40	42	44	46	48	50	52	54	56	58	60	62	64	66	68	70
53.0	2.17	2.16	2.15	2.14	2.12	2.10	2.08	2.06	2.04	2.01	1.98	1.95	1.92	1.88	1.85	1.81	1.77	1.72	1.68	1.63	1.58	1.53	1.48	1.42	1.36	1.30	1.24
54.0	2.27	2.26	2.25	2.23	2.22	2.20	2.18	2.16	2.13	2.11	2.08	2.05	2.01	1.98	1.94	1.90	1.86	1.82	1.77	1.72	1.68	1.62	1.57	1.51	1.46	1.39	1.33
55.0	2.36	2.35	2.34	2.33	2.31	2.29	2.27	2.25	2.23	2.20	2.17	2.14	2.11	2.07	2.04	2.00	1.96	1.91	1.87	1.82	1.77	1.72	1.67	1.61	1.55	1.49	1.43
56.0	2.46	2.45	2.44	2.42	2.41	2.39	2.37	2.35	2.32	2.30	2.27	2.24	2.21	2.17	2.13	2.10	2.05	2.01	1.97	1.92	1.87	1.82	1.76	1.71	1.65	1.59	1.53
57.0	2.56	2.55	2.54	2.52	2.51	2.49	2.47	2.45	2.42	2.40	2.37	2.34	2.31	2.27	2.23	2.19	2.15	2.11	2.06	2.02	1.97	1.92	1.86	1.81	1.75	1.69	1.62
58.0	2.66	2.65	2.64	2.63	2.61	2.59	2.57	2.55	2.52	2.50	2.47	2.44	2.41	2.37	2.33	2.30	2.25	2.21	2.17	2.12	2.07	2.02	1.96	1.91	1.85	1.79	1.73
59.0	2.76	2.75	2.74	2.73	2.71	2.69	2.67	2.65	2.63	2.60	2.57	2.54	2.51	2.47	2.44	2.40	2.36	2.31	2.27	2.22	2.17	2.12	2.07	2.01	1.95	1.89	1.83
60.0	2.87	2.86	2.85	2.83	2.82	2.80	2.78	2.76	2.73	2.71	2.68	2.65	2.61	2.58	2.54	2.50	2.46	2.42	2.37	2.33	2.28	2.22	2.17	2.11	2.06	2.00	1.93
61.0	2.97	2.96	2.95	2.94	2.92	2.90	2.88	2.86	2.84	2.81	2.78	2.75	2.72	2.69	2.65	2.61	2.57	2.52	2.48	2.43	2.38	2.33	2.28	2.22	2.16	2.10	2.04
62.0	3.08	3.07	3.06	3.05	3.03	3.01	2.99	2.97	2.95	2.92	2.89	2.86	2.83	2.79	2.76	2.72	2.68	2.63	2.59	2.54	2.49	2.44	2.38	2.33	2.27	2.21	2.15
63.0	3.19	3.18	3.17	3.16	3.14	3.12	3.10	3.08	3.06	3.03	3.00	2.97	2.94	2.90	2.87	2.83	2.79	2.74	2.70	2.65	2.60	2.55	2.49	2.44	2.38	2.32	2.26
64.0	3.30	3.29	3.28	3.27	3.25	3.23	3.21	3.19	3.17	3.14	3.11	3.08	3.05	3.01	2.98	2.94	2.90	2.85	2.81	2.76	2.71	2.66	2.61	2.55	2.49	2.43	2.37
65.0	3.42	3.41	3.39	3.38	3.37	3.35	3.33	3.30	3.28	3.25	3.23	3.20	3.16	3.13	3.09	3.05	3.01	2.97	2.92	2.87	2.82	2.77	2.72	2.66	2.60	2.54	2.48
66.0	3.53	3.52	3.51	3.50	3.48	3.46	3.44	3.42	3.40	3.37	3.34	3.31	3.28	3.24	3.21	3.17	3.13	3.08	3.04	2.99	2.94	2.89	2.83	2.78	2.72	2.66	2.60
67.0	3.65	3.64	3.63	3.61	3.60	3.58	3.56	3.54	3.51	3.49	3.46	3.43	3.39	3.36	3.32	3.28	3.24	3.20	3.15	3.11	3.06	3.00	2.95	2.89	2.84	2.78	2.71
68.0	3.77	3.76	3.74	3.73	3.72	3.70	3.68	3.66	3.63	3.60	3.58	3.55	3.51	3.48	3.44	3.40	3.36	3.32	3.27	3.22	3.17	3.12	3.07	3.01	2.95	2.89	2.83
69.0	3.89	3.88	3.86	3.85	3.84	3.82	3.80	3.78	3.75	3.72	3.70	3.67	3.63	3.60	3.56	3.52	3.48	3.44	3.39	3.34	3.29	3.24	3.19	3.13	3.07	3.01	2.95
70.0	4.01	4.00	3.99	3.97	3.96	3.94	3.92	3.90	3.87	3.85	3.82	3.79	3.76	3.72	3.68	3.64	3.60	3.56	3.51	3.47	3.42	3.36	3.31	3.25	3.20	3.14	3.07
71.0	4.13	4.12	4.11	4.10	4.08	4.06	4.04	4.02	4.00	3.97	3.94	3.91	3.88	3.84	3.81	3.77	3.73	3.68	3.64	3.59	3.54	3.49	3.43	3.38	3.32	3.26	3.20
72.0	4.26	4.25	4.24	4.22	4.21	4.19	4.17	4.15	4.12	4.10	4.07	4.04	4.00	3.97	3.93	3.89	3.85	3.81	3.76	3.72	3.67	3.61	3.56	3.50	3.45	3.39	3.32

LLN for FVC (L) - African American Females - NHANES III

Height (Inches)	18	20	22	24	26	28	30	32	34	36	38	40	42	44	46	48	50	52	54	56	58	60	62	64	66	68	70
53.0	1.68	1.68	1.66	1.65	1.63	1.62	1.60	1.57	1.55	1.52	1.50	1.46	1.43	1.40	1.36	1.32	1.28	1.24	1.19	1.14	1.09	1.04	0.99	0.93	0.87	0.81	0.75
54.0	1.76	1.75	1.74	1.73	1.71	1.69	1.67	1.65	1.63	1.60	1.57	1.54	1.51	1.47	1.44	1.40	1.36	1.31	1.27	1.22	1.17	1.12	1.06	1.01	0.95	0.89	0.83
55.0	1.84	1.83	1.82	1.80	1.79	1.77	1.75	1.73	1.70	1.68	1.65	1.62	1.58	1.55	1.51	1.47	1.43	1.39	1.34	1.30	1.25	1.19	1.14	1.08	1.03	0.97	0.90
56.0	1.92	1.91	1.89	1.88	1.86	1.85	1.83	1.80	1.78	1.75	1.73	1.70	1.66	1.63	1.59	1.55	1.51	1.47	1.42	1.37	1.32	1.27	1.22	1.16	1.10	1.04	0.98
57.0	1.99	1.99	1.97	1.96	1.94	1.93	1.91	1.88	1.86	1.83	1.81	1.77	1.74	1.71	1.67	1.63	1.59	1.55	1.50	1.45	1.40	1.35	1.30	1.24	1.18	1.12	1.06
58.0	2.08	2.07	2.05	2.04	2.03	2.01	1.99	1.97	1.94	1.91	1.89	1.86	1.82	1.79	1.75	1.71	1.67	1.63	1.58	1.53	1.48	1.43	1.38	1.32	1.26	1.20	1.14
59.0	2.16	2.15	2.14	2.12	2.11	2.09	2.07	2.05	2.02	2.00	1.97	1.94	1.91	1.87	1.83	1.79	1.75	1.71	1.66	1.62	1.57	1.52	1.46	1.41	1.35	1.29	1.22
60.0	2.24	2.23	2.22	2.21	2.19	2.17	2.15	2.13	2.11	2.08	2.05	2.02	1.99	1.95	1.92	1.88	1.84	1.79	1.75	1.70	1.65	1.60	1.55	1.49	1.43	1.37	1.31
61.0	2.33	2.32	2.31	2.29	2.28	2.26	2.24	2.22	2.19	2.17	2.14	2.11	2.07	2.04	2.00	1.96	1.92	1.88	1.83	1.79	1.74	1.68	1.63	1.57	1.52	1.46	1.39
62.0	2.41	2.40	2.39	2.38	2.36	2.35	2.33	2.30	2.28	2.25	2.22	2.19	2.16	2.13	2.09	2.05	2.01	1.97	1.92	1.87	1.82	1.77	1.72	1.66	1.60	1.54	1.48
63.0	2.50	2.49	2.48	2.47	2.45	2.43	2.41	2.39	2.37	2.34	2.31	2.28	2.25	2.21	2.18	2.14	2.10	2.05	2.01	1.96	1.91	1.86	1.80	1.75	1.69	1.63	1.57
64.0	2.59	2.58	2.57	2.56	2.54	2.52	2.50	2.48	2.46	2.43	2.40	2.37	2.34	2.30	2.27	2.23	2.19	2.14	2.10	2.05	2.00	1.95	1.89	1.84	1.78	1.72	1.66
65.0	2.68	2.67	2.66	2.65	2.63	2.61	2.59	2.57	2.55	2.52	2.49	2.46	2.43	2.39	2.36	2.32	2.28	2.23	2.19	2.14	2.09	2.04	1.99	1.93	1.87	1.81	1.75
66.0	2.77	2.77	2.75	2.74	2.72	2.71	2.69	2.66	2.64	2.61	2.58	2.55	2.52	2.49	2.45	2.41	2.37	2.33	2.28	2.23	2.18	2.13	2.08	2.02	1.96	1.90	1.84
67.0	2.87	2.86	2.85	2.83	2.82	2.80	2.78	2.76	2.73	2.71	2.68	2.65	2.62	2.58	2.54	2.50	2.46	2.42	2.37	2.33	2.28	2.23	2.17	2.12	2.06	2.00	1.93
68.0	2.96	2.95	2.94	2.93	2.91	2.89	2.87	2.85	2.83	2.80	2.77	2.74	2.71	2.68	2.64	2.60	2.56	2.51	2.47	2.42	2.37	2.32	2.27	2.21	2.15	2.09	2.03
69.0	3.06	3.05	3.04	3.03	3.01	2.99	2.97	2.95	2.92	2.90	2.87	2.84	2.81	2.77	2.73	2.70	2.65	2.61	2.57	2.52	2.47	2.42	2.36	2.31	2.25	2.19	2.13
70.0	3.16	3.15	3.14	3.12	3.11	3.09	3.07	3.05	3.02	3.00	2.97	2.94	2.90	2.87	2.83	2.79	2.75	2.71	2.66	2.62	2.57	2.51	2.46	2.40	2.35	2.29	2.22
71.0	3.26	3.25	3.24	3.22	3.21	3.19	3.17	3.15	3.12	3.10	3.07	3.04	3.00	2.97	2.93	2.89	2.85	2.81	2.76	2.72	2.67	2.61	2.56	2.50	2.45	2.39	2.32
72.0	3.36	3.35	3.34	3.32	3.31	3.29	3.27	3.25	3.22	3.20	3.17	3.14	3.10	3.07	3.03	2.99	2.95	2.91	2.86	2.82	2.77	2.71	2.66	2.60	2.55	2.49	2.42

Predicted FEV$_1$ (L) - African American Females - NHANES III

Height (Inches)	18	20	22	24	26	28	30	32	34	36	38	40	42	44	46	48	50	52	54	56	58	60	62	64	66	68	70
53.0	2.05	2.01	1.98	1.95	1.91	1.87	1.84	1.80	1.76	1.72	1.68	1.64	1.60	1.56	1.51	1.47	1.42	1.38	1.33	1.29	1.24	1.19	1.14	1.09	1.04	0.99	0.94
54.0	2.12	2.09	2.05	2.02	1.98	1.95	1.91	1.87	1.84	1.80	1.76	1.72	1.67	1.63	1.59	1.54	1.50	1.45	1.41	1.36	1.31	1.26	1.22	1.17	1.11	1.06	1.01
55.0	2.20	2.16	2.13	2.10	2.06	2.02	1.99	1.95	1.91	1.87	1.83	1.79	1.75	1.71	1.66	1.62	1.58	1.53	1.48	1.44	1.39	1.34	1.29	1.24	1.19	1.14	1.09
56.0	2.28	2.24	2.21	2.17	2.14	2.10	2.07	2.03	1.99	1.95	1.91	1.87	1.83	1.79	1.74	1.70	1.65	1.61	1.56	1.52	1.47	1.42	1.37	1.32	1.27	1.22	1.16
57.0	2.35	2.32	2.29	2.25	2.22	2.18	2.14	2.11	2.07	2.03	1.99	1.95	1.91	1.86	1.82	1.78	1.73	1.69	1.64	1.59	1.55	1.50	1.45	1.40	1.35	1.30	1.24
58.0	2.43	2.40	2.37	2.33	2.30	2.26	2.23	2.19	2.15	2.11	2.07	2.03	1.99	1.94	1.90	1.86	1.81	1.77	1.72	1.67	1.63	1.58	1.53	1.48	1.43	1.38	1.32
59.0	2.52	2.48	2.45	2.42	2.38	2.34	2.31	2.27	2.23	2.19	2.15	2.11	2.07	2.03	1.98	1.94	1.90	1.85	1.80	1.76	1.71	1.66	1.61	1.56	1.51	1.46	1.41
60.0	2.60	2.57	2.53	2.50	2.46	2.43	2.39	2.35	2.31	2.27	2.23	2.19	2.15	2.11	2.07	2.02	1.98	1.93	1.89	1.84	1.79	1.74	1.69	1.64	1.59	1.54	1.49
61.0	2.68	2.65	2.62	2.58	2.55	2.51	2.47	2.44	2.40	2.36	2.32	2.28	2.24	2.19	2.15	2.11	2.06	2.02	1.97	1.92	1.88	1.83	1.78	1.73	1.68	1.63	1.57
62.0	2.77	2.74	2.70	2.67	2.63	2.60	2.56	2.52	2.48	2.45	2.41	2.36	2.32	2.28	2.24	2.19	2.15	2.10	2.06	2.01	1.96	1.91	1.86	1.81	1.76	1.71	1.66
63.0	2.86	2.83	2.79	2.76	2.72	2.69	2.65	2.61	2.57	2.53	2.49	2.45	2.41	2.37	2.33	2.28	2.24	2.19	2.14	2.10	2.05	2.00	1.95	1.90	1.85	1.80	1.75
64.0	2.95	2.91	2.88	2.85	2.81	2.77	2.74	2.70	2.66	2.62	2.58	2.54	2.50	2.46	2.41	2.37	2.33	2.28	2.23	2.19	2.14	2.09	2.04	1.99	1.94	1.89	1.84
65.0	3.04	3.00	2.97	2.94	2.90	2.86	2.83	2.79	2.75	2.71	2.67	2.63	2.59	2.55	2.50	2.46	2.42	2.37	2.32	2.28	2.23	2.18	2.13	2.08	2.03	1.98	1.93
66.0	3.13	3.10	3.06	3.03	2.99	2.96	2.92	2.88	2.84	2.80	2.76	2.72	2.68	2.64	2.60	2.55	2.51	2.46	2.42	2.37	2.32	2.27	2.22	2.17	2.12	2.07	2.02
67.0	3.22	3.19	3.16	3.12	3.09	3.05	3.01	2.97	2.94	2.90	2.86	2.82	2.77	2.73	2.69	2.65	2.60	2.55	2.51	2.46	2.41	2.37	2.32	2.27	2.22	2.16	2.11
68.0	3.32	3.28	3.25	3.22	3.18	3.14	3.11	3.07	3.03	2.99	2.95	2.91	2.87	2.83	2.78	2.74	2.69	2.65	2.60	2.56	2.51	2.46	2.41	2.36	2.31	2.26	2.21
69.0	3.41	3.38	3.35	3.31	3.28	3.24	3.20	3.16	3.13	3.09	3.05	3.01	2.96	2.92	2.88	2.84	2.79	2.75	2.70	2.65	2.60	2.56	2.51	2.46	2.41	2.35	2.30
70.0	3.51	3.48	3.44	3.41	3.37	3.34	3.30	3.26	3.22	3.18	3.14	3.10	3.06	3.02	2.98	2.93	2.89	2.84	2.80	2.75	2.70	2.65	2.60	2.55	2.50	2.45	2.40
71.0	3.61	3.58	3.54	3.51	3.47	3.44	3.40	3.36	3.32	3.28	3.24	3.20	3.16	3.12	3.08	3.03	2.99	2.94	2.90	2.85	2.80	2.75	2.70	2.65	2.60	2.55	2.50
72.0	3.71	3.68	3.64	3.61	3.57	3.54	3.50	3.46	3.42	3.38	3.34	3.30	3.26	3.22	3.18	3.13	3.09	3.04	3.00	2.95	2.90	2.85	2.80	2.75	2.70	2.65	2.60

LLN for FEV$_1$ (L) - African American Females - NHANES III

Height (Inches)	18	20	22	24	26	28	30	32	34	36	38	40	42	44	46	48	50	52	54	56	58	60	62	64	66	68	70
53.0	1.63	1.60	1.56	1.53	1.49	1.46	1.42	1.38	1.34	1.30	1.26	1.22	1.18	1.14	1.10	1.05	1.01	0.96	0.92	0.87	0.82	0.77	0.72	0.67	0.62	0.57	0.52
54.0	1.69	1.66	1.62	1.59	1.55	1.52	1.48	1.44	1.40	1.36	1.32	1.28	1.24	1.20	1.16	1.11	1.07	1.02	0.98	0.93	0.88	0.83	0.78	0.73	0.68	0.63	0.58
55.0	1.75	1.72	1.68	1.65	1.61	1.58	1.54	1.50	1.46	1.42	1.38	1.34	1.30	1.26	1.22	1.17	1.13	1.08	1.04	0.99	0.94	0.89	0.84	0.79	0.74	0.69	0.64
56.0	1.81	1.78	1.74	1.71	1.67	1.64	1.60	1.56	1.52	1.48	1.44	1.40	1.36	1.32	1.28	1.23	1.19	1.14	1.10	1.05	1.00	0.95	0.90	0.85	0.80	0.75	0.70
57.0	1.87	1.84	1.81	1.77	1.74	1.70	1.66	1.62	1.59	1.55	1.51	1.47	1.42	1.38	1.34	1.30	1.25	1.21	1.16	1.11	1.06	1.02	0.97	0.92	0.87	0.81	0.76
58.0	1.94	1.90	1.87	1.83	1.80	1.76	1.73	1.69	1.65	1.61	1.57	1.53	1.49	1.45	1.40	1.36	1.31	1.27	1.22	1.18	1.13	1.08	1.03	0.98	0.93	0.88	0.82
59.0	2.00	1.97	1.93	1.90	1.86	1.83	1.79	1.75	1.71	1.67	1.63	1.59	1.55	1.51	1.47	1.42	1.38	1.33	1.29	1.24	1.19	1.14	1.09	1.04	0.99	0.94	0.89
60.0	2.07	2.03	2.00	1.96	1.93	1.89	1.86	1.82	1.78	1.74	1.70	1.66	1.62	1.58	1.53	1.49	1.44	1.40	1.35	1.31	1.26	1.21	1.16	1.11	1.06	1.01	0.95
61.0	2.13	2.10	2.07	2.03	2.00	1.96	1.92	1.88	1.85	1.81	1.77	1.73	1.68	1.64	1.60	1.56	1.51	1.47	1.42	1.37	1.32	1.28	1.23	1.18	1.13	1.07	1.02
62.0	2.20	2.17	2.13	2.10	2.06	2.03	1.99	1.95	1.91	1.88	1.84	1.79	1.75	1.71	1.67	1.62	1.58	1.53	1.49	1.44	1.39	1.34	1.29	1.24	1.19	1.14	1.09
63.0	2.27	2.24	2.20	2.17	2.13	2.10	2.06	2.02	1.98	1.94	1.90	1.86	1.82	1.78	1.74	1.69	1.65	1.60	1.56	1.51	1.46	1.41	1.36	1.31	1.26	1.21	1.16
64.0	2.34	2.31	2.27	2.24	2.20	2.17	2.13	2.09	2.05	2.01	1.97	1.93	1.89	1.85	1.81	1.76	1.72	1.67	1.63	1.58	1.53	1.48	1.43	1.38	1.33	1.28	1.23
65.0	2.41	2.38	2.34	2.31	2.27	2.24	2.20	2.16	2.12	2.09	2.05	2.00	1.96	1.92	1.88	1.83	1.79	1.74	1.70	1.65	1.60	1.55	1.50	1.45	1.40	1.35	1.30
66.0	2.48	2.45	2.42	2.38	2.35	2.31	2.27	2.24	2.20	2.16	2.12	2.08	2.04	1.99	1.95	1.91	1.86	1.82	1.77	1.72	1.67	1.63	1.58	1.53	1.48	1.42	1.37
67.0	2.56	2.52	2.49	2.45	2.42	2.38	2.35	2.31	2.27	2.23	2.19	2.15	2.11	2.07	2.02	1.98	1.93	1.89	1.84	1.80	1.75	1.70	1.65	1.60	1.55	1.50	1.44
68.0	2.63	2.60	2.56	2.53	2.49	2.46	2.42	2.38	2.34	2.31	2.27	2.22	2.18	2.14	2.10	2.05	2.01	1.96	1.92	1.87	1.82	1.77	1.72	1.67	1.62	1.57	1.52
69.0	2.71	2.67	2.64	2.60	2.57	2.53	2.50	2.46	2.42	2.38	2.34	2.30	2.26	2.22	2.17	2.13	2.08	2.04	1.99	1.95	1.90	1.85	1.80	1.75	1.70	1.65	1.59
70.0	2.78	2.75	2.72	2.68	2.65	2.61	2.57	2.54	2.50	2.46	2.42	2.38	2.33	2.29	2.25	2.21	2.16	2.12	2.07	2.02	1.97	1.93	1.88	1.83	1.78	1.72	1.67
71.0	2.86	2.83	2.79	2.76	2.72	2.69	2.65	2.61	2.57	2.54	2.50	2.45	2.41	2.37	2.33	2.28	2.24	2.19	2.15	2.10	2.05	2.00	1.95	1.90	1.85	1.80	1.75
72.0	2.94	2.91	2.87	2.84	2.80	2.77	2.73	2.69	2.65	2.61	2.57	2.53	2.49	2.45	2.41	2.36	2.32	2.27	2.23	2.18	2.13	2.08	2.03	1.98	1.93	1.88	1.83

Predicted FVC (L) - Mexican American Females - NHANES III

Height (Inches)	Age																											
	18	20	22	24	26	28	30	32	34	36	38	40	42	44	46	48	50	52	54	56	58	60	62	64	66	68	70
53.0	2.68	2.67	2.66	2.64	2.62	2.60	2.58	2.56	2.53	2.51	2.48	2.45	2.41	2.38	2.34	2.30	2.26	2.22	2.18	2.13	2.08	2.03	1.98	1.93	1.87	1.82	1.76
54.0	2.78	2.77	2.75	2.74	2.72	2.70	2.68	2.66	2.63	2.60	2.58	2.54	2.51	2.48	2.44	2.40	2.36	2.32	2.28	2.23	2.18	2.13	2.08	2.03	1.97	1.91	1.85
55.0	2.88	2.87	2.85	2.84	2.82	2.80	2.78	2.76	2.73	2.70	2.68	2.64	2.61	2.58	2.54	2.50	2.46	2.42	2.38	2.33	2.28	2.23	2.18	2.13	2.07	2.01	1.95
56.0	2.98	2.97	2.96	2.94	2.92	2.90	2.88	2.86	2.83	2.81	2.78	2.75	2.71	2.68	2.64	2.60	2.56	2.52	2.48	2.43	2.38	2.33	2.28	2.23	2.17	2.12	2.06
57.0	3.09	3.07	3.06	3.04	3.03	3.01	2.99	2.96	2.94	2.91	2.88	2.85	2.82	2.78	2.75	2.71	2.67	2.63	2.58	2.54	2.49	2.44	2.39	2.33	2.28	2.22	2.16
58.0	3.19	3.18	3.17	3.15	3.13	3.11	3.09	3.07	3.04	3.02	2.99	2.96	2.92	2.89	2.85	2.81	2.77	2.73	2.69	2.64	2.59	2.54	2.49	2.44	2.38	2.33	2.27
59.0	3.30	3.29	3.27	3.26	3.24	3.22	3.20	3.18	3.15	3.12	3.09	3.06	3.03	3.00	2.96	2.92	2.88	2.84	2.80	2.75	2.70	2.65	2.60	2.55	2.49	2.43	2.37
60.0	3.41	3.40	3.38	3.37	3.35	3.33	3.31	3.29	3.26	3.23	3.20	3.17	3.14	3.11	3.07	3.03	2.99	2.95	2.90	2.86	2.81	2.76	2.71	2.66	2.60	2.54	2.48
61.0	3.52	3.51	3.49	3.48	3.46	3.44	3.42	3.40	3.37	3.34	3.32	3.28	3.25	3.22	3.18	3.14	3.10	3.06	3.02	2.97	2.92	2.87	2.82	2.77	2.71	2.65	2.59
62.0	3.63	3.62	3.61	3.59	3.57	3.55	3.53	3.51	3.48	3.46	3.43	3.40	3.36	3.33	3.29	3.26	3.22	3.17	3.13	3.08	3.03	2.99	2.93	2.88	2.82	2.77	2.71
63.0	3.75	3.74	3.72	3.71	3.69	3.67	3.65	3.62	3.60	3.57	3.54	3.51	3.48	3.45	3.41	3.37	3.33	3.29	3.24	3.20	3.15	3.10	3.05	2.99	2.94	2.88	2.82
64.0	3.86	3.85	3.84	3.82	3.81	3.79	3.76	3.74	3.72	3.69	3.66	3.63	3.60	3.56	3.53	3.49	3.45	3.40	3.36	3.31	3.27	3.22	3.16	3.11	3.06	3.00	2.94
65.0	3.98	3.97	3.96	3.94	3.92	3.90	3.88	3.86	3.83	3.81	3.78	3.75	3.72	3.68	3.64	3.61	3.57	3.52	3.48	3.43	3.38	3.34	3.28	3.23	3.17	3.12	3.06
66.0	4.10	4.09	4.08	4.06	4.04	4.02	4.00	3.98	3.95	3.93	3.90	3.87	3.84	3.80	3.76	3.73	3.69	3.64	3.60	3.55	3.51	3.46	3.40	3.35	3.29	3.24	3.18
67.0	4.23	4.21	4.20	4.18	4.17	4.15	4.13	4.10	4.08	4.05	4.02	3.99	3.96	3.92	3.89	3.85	3.81	3.77	3.72	3.68	3.63	3.58	3.53	3.47	3.42	3.36	3.30
68.0	4.35	4.34	4.32	4.31	4.29	4.27	4.25	4.23	4.20	4.17	4.15	4.11	4.08	4.05	4.01	3.97	3.93	3.89	3.85	3.80	3.75	3.70	3.65	3.60	3.54	3.48	3.42
69.0	4.48	4.46	4.45	4.43	4.42	4.40	4.38	4.35	4.33	4.30	4.27	4.24	4.21	4.17	4.14	4.10	4.06	4.02	3.97	3.93	3.88	3.83	3.78	3.72	3.67	3.61	3.55

LLN for FVC (L) - Mexican American Females - NHANES III

Height (Inches)	Age																											
	18	20	22	24	26	28	30	32	34	36	38	40	42	44	46	48	50	52	54	56	58	60	62	64	66	68	70
53.0	2.20	2.18	2.17	2.15	2.14	2.12	2.10	2.07	2.05	2.02	1.99	1.96	1.93	1.89	1.86	1.82	1.78	1.74	1.69	1.65	1.60	1.55	1.50	1.44	1.39	1.33	1.27
54.0	2.28	2.26	2.25	2.23	2.22	2.20	2.18	2.15	2.13	2.10	2.07	2.04	2.01	1.97	1.94	1.90	1.86	1.82	1.77	1.73	1.68	1.63	1.58	1.52	1.47	1.41	1.35
55.0	2.36	2.35	2.33	2.32	2.30	2.28	2.26	2.23	2.21	2.18	2.15	2.12	2.09	2.06	2.02	1.98	1.94	1.90	1.85	1.81	1.76	1.71	1.66	1.60	1.55	1.49	1.43
56.0	2.44	2.43	2.41	2.40	2.38	2.36	2.34	2.32	2.29	2.27	2.24	2.21	2.17	2.14	2.10	2.06	2.02	1.98	1.94	1.89	1.84	1.79	1.74	1.69	1.63	1.57	1.52
57.0	2.52	2.51	2.50	2.48	2.47	2.45	2.43	2.40	2.38	2.35	2.32	2.29	2.26	2.22	2.19	2.15	2.11	2.07	2.02	1.97	1.93	1.88	1.83	1.77	1.72	1.66	1.60
58.0	2.61	2.60	2.58	2.57	2.55	2.53	2.51	2.49	2.46	2.44	2.41	2.38	2.34	2.31	2.27	2.23	2.19	2.15	2.11	2.06	2.01	1.96	1.91	1.86	1.80	1.74	1.69
59.0	2.70	2.69	2.67	2.66	2.64	2.62	2.60	2.57	2.55	2.52	2.49	2.46	2.43	2.40	2.36	2.32	2.28	2.24	2.19	2.15	2.10	2.05	2.00	1.95	1.89	1.83	1.77
60.0	2.79	2.77	2.76	2.75	2.73	2.71	2.69	2.66	2.64	2.61	2.58	2.55	2.52	2.48	2.45	2.41	2.37	2.33	2.28	2.24	2.19	2.14	2.09	2.03	1.98	1.92	1.86
61.0	2.88	2.87	2.85	2.84	2.82	2.80	2.78	2.75	2.73	2.70	2.67	2.64	2.61	2.57	2.54	2.50	2.46	2.42	2.37	2.33	2.28	2.23	2.18	2.12	2.07	2.01	1.95
62.0	2.97	2.96	2.94	2.93	2.91	2.89	2.87	2.85	2.82	2.79	2.76	2.73	2.70	2.67	2.63	2.59	2.55	2.51	2.47	2.42	2.37	2.32	2.27	2.22	2.16	2.10	2.04
63.0	3.06	3.05	3.04	3.02	3.00	2.98	2.96	2.94	2.91	2.89	2.86	2.83	2.79	2.76	2.72	2.68	2.64	2.60	2.56	2.51	2.46	2.41	2.36	2.31	2.25	2.20	2.14
64.0	3.16	3.15	3.13	3.12	3.10	3.08	3.06	3.03	3.01	2.98	2.95	2.92	2.89	2.85	2.82	2.78	2.74	2.70	2.65	2.61	2.56	2.51	2.46	2.40	2.35	2.29	2.23
65.0	3.25	3.24	3.23	3.21	3.19	3.17	3.15	3.13	3.11	3.08	3.05	3.02	2.99	2.95	2.91	2.88	2.84	2.79	2.75	2.70	2.66	2.61	2.55	2.50	2.44	2.39	2.33
66.0	3.35	3.34	3.33	3.31	3.29	3.27	3.25	3.23	3.20	3.18	3.15	3.12	3.08	3.05	3.01	2.97	2.93	2.89	2.85	2.80	2.75	2.70	2.65	2.60	2.54	2.49	2.43
67.0	3.45	3.44	3.42	3.41	3.39	3.37	3.35	3.33	3.30	3.28	3.25	3.22	3.18	3.15	3.11	3.07	3.03	2.99	2.95	2.90	2.85	2.80	2.75	2.70	2.64	2.58	2.53
68.0	3.55	3.54	3.53	3.51	3.49	3.47	3.45	3.43	3.40	3.38	3.35	3.32	3.28	3.25	3.21	3.17	3.13	3.09	3.05	3.00	2.95	2.90	2.85	2.80	2.74	2.69	2.63
69.0	3.65	3.64	3.63	3.61	3.59	3.58	3.55	3.53	3.51	3.48	3.45	3.42	3.39	3.35	3.31	3.28	3.24	3.19	3.15	3.10	3.06	3.01	2.95	2.90	2.85	2.79	2.73

Predicted FEV$_1$ (L) - Mexican American Females - NHANES III

Height (Inches)	18	20	22	24	26	28	30	32	34	36	38	40	42	44	46	48	50	52	54	56	58	60	62	64	66	68	70
53.0	2.41	2.37	2.34	2.31	2.27	2.24	2.20	2.16	2.12	2.08	2.04	2.00	1.96	1.92	1.87	1.83	1.78	1.74	1.69	1.64	1.59	1.54	1.49	1.44	1.39	1.33	1.28
54.0	2.49	2.46	2.43	2.39	2.36	2.32	2.28	2.25	2.21	2.17	2.13	2.09	2.05	2.00	1.96	1.91	1.87	1.82	1.77	1.73	1.68	1.63	1.57	1.52	1.47	1.42	1.36
55.0	2.58	2.54	2.51	2.48	2.44	2.41	2.37	2.33	2.29	2.25	2.21	2.17	2.13	2.09	2.04	2.00	1.95	1.91	1.86	1.81	1.76	1.71	1.66	1.61	1.56	1.50	1.45
56.0	2.66	2.63	2.60	2.56	2.53	2.49	2.46	2.42	2.38	2.34	2.30	2.26	2.22	2.17	2.13	2.09	2.04	1.99	1.95	1.90	1.85	1.80	1.75	1.70	1.64	1.59	1.53
57.0	2.75	2.72	2.69	2.65	2.62	2.58	2.55	2.51	2.47	2.43	2.39	2.35	2.31	2.26	2.22	2.17	2.13	2.08	2.03	1.99	1.94	1.89	1.84	1.78	1.73	1.68	1.62
58.0	2.84	2.81	2.78	2.74	2.71	2.67	2.64	2.60	2.56	2.52	2.48	2.44	2.40	2.35	2.31	2.26	2.22	2.17	2.13	2.08	2.03	1.98	1.93	1.87	1.82	1.77	1.71
59.0	2.93	2.90	2.87	2.83	2.80	2.76	2.73	2.69	2.65	2.61	2.57	2.53	2.49	2.45	2.40	2.36	2.31	2.26	2.22	2.17	2.12	2.07	2.02	1.97	1.91	1.86	1.80
60.0	3.03	2.99	2.96	2.93	2.89	2.86	2.82	2.78	2.74	2.71	2.66	2.62	2.58	2.54	2.49	2.45	2.40	2.36	2.31	2.26	2.21	2.16	2.11	2.06	2.01	1.95	1.90
61.0	3.12	3.09	3.06	3.02	2.99	2.95	2.92	2.88	2.84	2.80	2.76	2.72	2.68	2.63	2.59	2.54	2.50	2.45	2.41	2.36	2.31	2.26	2.21	2.15	2.10	2.05	1.99
62.0	3.22	3.19	3.15	3.12	3.08	3.05	3.01	2.97	2.94	2.90	2.86	2.82	2.77	2.73	2.69	2.64	2.60	2.55	2.50	2.45	2.40	2.35	2.30	2.25	2.20	2.14	2.09
63.0	3.32	3.28	3.25	3.22	3.18	3.15	3.11	3.07	3.03	2.99	2.95	2.91	2.87	2.83	2.78	2.74	2.69	2.65	2.60	2.55	2.50	2.45	2.40	2.35	2.30	2.24	2.19
64.0	3.42	3.38	3.35	3.32	3.28	3.25	3.21	3.17	3.13	3.09	3.05	3.01	2.97	2.93	2.88	2.84	2.79	2.75	2.70	2.65	2.60	2.55	2.50	2.45	2.39	2.34	2.29
65.0	3.52	3.49	3.45	3.42	3.38	3.35	3.31	3.27	3.23	3.20	3.16	3.11	3.07	3.03	2.98	2.94	2.89	2.85	2.80	2.75	2.70	2.65	2.60	2.55	2.50	2.44	2.39
66.0	3.62	3.59	3.55	3.52	3.49	3.45	3.41	3.38	3.34	3.30	3.26	3.22	3.17	3.13	3.09	3.04	3.00	2.95	2.90	2.85	2.81	2.75	2.70	2.65	2.60	2.55	2.49
67.0	3.72	3.69	3.66	3.63	3.59	3.55	3.52	3.48	3.44	3.40	3.36	3.32	3.28	3.24	3.19	3.15	3.10	3.05	3.01	2.96	2.91	2.86	2.81	2.76	2.70	2.65	2.59
68.0	3.83	3.80	3.76	3.73	3.70	3.66	3.62	3.59	3.55	3.51	3.47	3.43	3.38	3.34	3.30	3.25	3.21	3.16	3.11	3.06	3.02	2.97	2.91	2.86	2.81	2.76	2.70
69.0	3.94	3.91	3.87	3.84	3.80	3.77	3.73	3.69	3.65	3.62	3.58	3.53	3.49	3.45	3.41	3.36	3.31	3.27	3.22	3.17	3.12	3.07	3.02	2.97	2.92	2.86	2.81

LLN for FEV$_1$ (L) - Mexican American Females - NHANES III

Height (Inches)	18	20	22	24	26	28	30	32	34	36	38	40	42	44	46	48	50	52	54	56	58	60	62	64	66	68	70
53.0	2.00	1.96	1.93	1.90	1.86	1.83	1.79	1.75	1.71	1.67	1.63	1.59	1.55	1.51	1.46	1.42	1.37	1.33	1.28	1.23	1.18	1.13	1.08	1.03	0.98	0.92	0.87
54.0	2.06	2.03	2.00	1.97	1.93	1.90	1.86	1.82	1.78	1.74	1.70	1.66	1.62	1.58	1.53	1.49	1.44	1.40	1.35	1.30	1.25	1.20	1.15	1.10	1.04	0.99	0.94
55.0	2.13	2.10	2.07	2.04	2.00	1.96	1.93	1.89	1.85	1.81	1.77	1.73	1.69	1.65	1.60	1.56	1.51	1.46	1.42	1.37	1.32	1.27	1.22	1.17	1.11	1.06	1.00
56.0	2.21	2.17	2.14	2.11	2.07	2.04	2.00	1.96	1.92	1.88	1.84	1.80	1.76	1.72	1.67	1.63	1.58	1.54	1.49	1.44	1.39	1.34	1.29	1.24	1.18	1.13	1.08
57.0	2.28	2.25	2.21	2.18	2.14	2.11	2.07	2.03	1.99	1.96	1.92	1.87	1.83	1.79	1.74	1.70	1.65	1.61	1.56	1.51	1.46	1.41	1.36	1.31	1.26	1.20	1.15
58.0	2.35	2.32	2.29	2.25	2.22	2.18	2.14	2.11	2.07	2.03	1.99	1.95	1.91	1.86	1.82	1.77	1.73	1.68	1.63	1.59	1.54	1.49	1.43	1.38	1.33	1.28	1.22
59.0	2.43	2.39	2.36	2.33	2.29	2.26	2.22	2.18	2.14	2.10	2.06	2.02	1.98	1.94	1.89	1.85	1.80	1.76	1.71	1.66	1.61	1.56	1.51	1.46	1.40	1.35	1.30
60.0	2.50	2.47	2.44	2.40	2.37	2.33	2.29	2.26	2.22	2.18	2.14	2.10	2.06	2.01	1.97	1.92	1.88	1.83	1.78	1.74	1.69	1.64	1.59	1.53	1.48	1.43	1.37
61.0	2.58	2.55	2.51	2.48	2.44	2.41	2.37	2.33	2.30	2.26	2.22	2.18	2.13	2.09	2.05	2.00	1.96	1.91	1.86	1.81	1.76	1.71	1.66	1.61	1.56	1.50	1.45
62.0	2.66	2.62	2.59	2.56	2.52	2.49	2.45	2.41	2.37	2.34	2.29	2.25	2.21	2.17	2.12	2.08	2.03	1.99	1.94	1.89	1.84	1.79	1.74	1.69	1.64	1.58	1.53
63.0	2.74	2.70	2.67	2.64	2.60	2.57	2.53	2.49	2.45	2.41	2.37	2.33	2.29	2.25	2.20	2.16	2.11	2.07	2.02	1.97	1.92	1.87	1.82	1.77	1.72	1.66	1.61
64.0	2.82	2.79	2.75	2.72	2.68	2.65	2.61	2.57	2.54	2.50	2.46	2.41	2.37	2.33	2.29	2.24	2.19	2.15	2.10	2.05	2.00	1.95	1.90	1.85	1.80	1.74	1.69
65.0	2.90	2.87	2.83	2.80	2.77	2.73	2.69	2.66	2.62	2.58	2.54	2.50	2.45	2.41	2.37	2.32	2.28	2.23	2.18	2.13	2.09	2.04	1.98	1.93	1.88	1.83	1.77
66.0	2.98	2.95	2.92	2.88	2.85	2.81	2.78	2.74	2.70	2.66	2.62	2.58	2.54	2.50	2.45	2.41	2.36	2.31	2.27	2.22	2.17	2.12	2.07	2.02	1.96	1.91	1.85
67.0	3.07	3.04	3.00	2.97	2.93	2.90	2.86	2.82	2.79	2.75	2.71	2.67	2.62	2.58	2.54	2.49	2.45	2.40	2.35	2.30	2.25	2.20	2.15	2.10	2.05	1.99	1.94
68.0	3.15	3.12	3.09	3.06	3.02	2.98	2.95	2.91	2.87	2.83	2.79	2.75	2.71	2.67	2.62	2.58	2.53	2.49	2.44	2.39	2.34	2.29	2.24	2.19	2.13	2.08	2.03
69.0	3.24	3.21	3.18	3.14	3.11	3.07	3.04	3.00	2.96	2.92	2.88	2.84	2.80	2.75	2.71	2.66	2.62	2.57	2.53	2.48	2.43	2.38	2.33	2.27	2.22	2.17	2.11

APPENDIX B

CHECKLIST FOR SPIROMETRY PROCEDURE MANUAL

✔ **That your spirometry procedure manual addresses OSHA recommendations on each of these topics:**

PERSONNEL TRAINING

- ☐ For PLHCPs: Completion of a NIOSH-approved spirometry course or equivalent training that emphasizes technical errors and correct interpretation of results (Section 2.1.1).

- ☐ For technicians and other persons conducting occupational spirometry tests: Completion of a NIOSH-approved course and periodic NIOSH-approved refresher courses (Section 2.1.1).

EQUIPMENT USE

- ☐ Equipment calibration check procedures and how often they are performed (Section 2.2.2).

- ☐ Protocols for periodic spirometer maintenance and for correcting common malfunctions (see manual for your particular spirometer).

- ☐ Protocols to prevent and/or correct sensor contamination and zero-flow errors in flow-type spirometers (Section 2.2.3).

- ☐ Instructions for infection control procedures, including cleaning or sterilizing the spirometer (Section 2.2.4).

CONDUCTING SPIROMETRY TESTS

- ☐ Pre-test eligibility questions (Section 2.3.1).

- ☐ Detailed spirometry testing protocol, including number of maneuvers to be attempted, criteria for acceptable start and end of test, repeatability criteria, criteria for saving/deleting curves, test posture, and noseclip use (Sections 2.3.1, 2.3.2, and 2.3.4).

- ☐ Information to be recorded on test reports, including test posture, subject effort, and technician ID (Section 6.0).

- ☐ List of necessary supplies.

CRITERIA FOR VALID TESTS AND REPORTING RESULTS

- [ ] Criteria for valid tests: at least 3 acceptable curves with repeatable FVC and FEV_1 (Section 2.3.4).
- [ ] Reporting of largest FVC and FEV_1, even if on different curves, and use of those values to compute FEV_1/FVC (Section 2.3.5).

REFERENCE VALUES AND INTERPRETATION ALGORITHMS

- [ ] Source of reference values ("predicted normals") and race-adjustment factors used (Sections 3.1.1 and 3.1.2).
- [ ] Spirometer interpretation algorithm used (Section 3.1.3).
- [ ] Spirometer configuration settings (Sections 2 and 3).

QA REVIEWS

- [ ] Protocol for QA reviews including frequency of sampling tests, criteria for inclusion in the QA sample, and name of designated QA reviewer (Section 4.0).

RECORDKEEPING

- [ ] Date and filename for the current version of the procedure manual (Section 6.0).
- [ ] Instructions to save each of the following (Section 6.0):
    - [ ] Sample report of worker test results.
    - [ ] All spirometer maintenance and calibration check records.
    - [ ] Manufacturer's spirometer user manual and contact information for manufacturer and local distributor.
    - [ ] Written verification from manufacturer that a prototype spirometer passed laboratory validation testing, meeting at least ATS/ERS minimum specifications for accuracy and precision (Section 2.2.1).
    - [ ] Personnel training certificates and evaluation records.

OSHA REGIONAL OFFICES

Region I
Boston Regional Office
(CT*, ME, MA, NH, RI, VT*)
JFK Federal Building, Room E340
Boston, MA 02203
(617) 565-9860 (617) 565-9827 Fax

Region II
New York Regional Office
(NJ*, NY*, PR*, VI*)
201 Varick Street, Room 670
New York, NY 10014
(212) 337-2378 (212) 337-2371 Fax

Region III
Philadelphia Regional Office
(DE, DC, MD*, PA, VA*, WV)
The Curtis Center
170 S. Independence Mall West
Suite 740 West
Philadelphia, PA 19106-3309
(215) 861-4900 (215) 861-4904 Fax

Region IV
Atlanta Regional Office
(AL, FL, GA, KY*, MS, NC*, SC*, TN*)
61 Forsyth Street, SW, Room 6T50
Atlanta, GA 30303
(678) 237-0400 (678) 237-0447 Fax

Region V
Chicago Regional Office
(IL*, IN*, MI*, MN*, OH, WI)
230 South Dearborn Street
Room 3244
Chicago, IL 60604
(312) 353-2220 (312) 353-7774 Fax

Region VI
Dallas Regional Office
(AR, LA, NM*, OK, TX)
525 Griffin Street, Room 602
Dallas, TX 75202
(972) 850-4145 (972) 850-4149 Fax
(972) 850-4150 FSO Fax

Region VII
Kansas City Regional Office
(IA*, KS, MO, NE)
Two Pershing Square Building
2300 Main Street, Suite 1010
Kansas City, MO 64108-2416
(816) 283-8745 (816) 283-0547 Fax

Region VIII
Denver Regional Office
(CO, MT, ND, SD, UT*, WY*)
Cesar Chavez Memorial Building
1244 Speer Boulevard, Suite 551
Denver, CO 80204
(720) 264-6550 (720) 264-6585 Fax

Region IX
San Francisco Regional Office
(AZ*, CA*, HI*, NV*, and American Samoa,
Guam and the Northern Mariana Islands)
90 7th Street, Suite 18100
San Francisco, CA 94103
(415) 625-2547 (415) 625-2534 Fax

Region X
Seattle Regional Office
(AK*, ID, OR*, WA*)
300 Fifth Avenue, Suite 1280
Seattle, WA 98104
(206) 757-6700 (206) 757-6705 Fax

*These states and territories operate their own OSHA-approved job safety and health plans and cover state and local government employees as well as private sector employees. The Connecticut, Illinois, New Jersey, New York and Virgin Islands programs cover public employees only. (Private sector workers in these states are covered by Federal OSHA). States with approved programs must have standards that are identical to, or at least as effective as, the Federal OSHA standards.

Note: To get contact information for OSHA area offices, OSHA-approved state plans and OSHA consultation projects, please visit us online at www.osha.gov or call us at 1-800-321-OSHA (6742).

HOW TO CONTACT OSHA

For questions or to get information or advice, to report an emergency, report a fatality or catastrophe, order publications, sign up for OSHA's e-newsletter *QuickTakes*, or to file a confidential complaint, contact your nearest OSHA office, visit www.osha.gov or call OSHA at 1-800-321-OSHA (6742), TTY 1-877-889-5627.

**For assistance, contact us.
We are OSHA. We can help.**

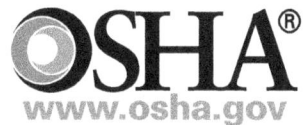

www.ingramcontent.com/pod-product-compliance
Lightning Source LLC
Chambersburg PA
CBHW081739170526
45167CB00009B/3878